# Smell the Rose

# Blow Out

# the Candle

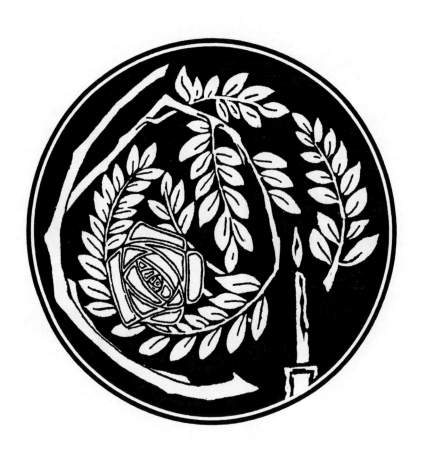

# Smell the Rose
# Blow Out
# the Candle

A personal story of coping
with sick lungs and
broken spirits by balancing
the mind-body-spirit
for wellness.

William R. Probstfield

This book was printed in the United States of America.

Cover medallion design by Lisa Drake

Author photo by Chere Jones

**To order additional copies of this book, contact:**
Xlibris Corporation
1-888-795-4274
www.Xlibris.com
Orders@Xlibris.com
18505

# Contents

Dedicated to my wife,

**Janet Alice**

a companion and caregiver
par excellence

and
Remembering
all my other COPD friends
who have gone on ahead of me.

# Acknowledgments

First of all, I thank Sandra and Larry, a couple of Northwest travelers, who seemed to have come to us as messengers with encouragement to write a book.

I would like to thank the many other people who encouraged me in this endeavor. Among them are my COPD Internet friends, Fran, Starion and Beej. Most of all, I thank my wife, Janet, my partner, supporter, first editor, caregiver and without whom I would not have attempted to put my thoughts in a book. Finally I express my appreciation to Koo and Yindee, my Siamese guys who have supported me every day for fourteen years. During the hundreds of hours I spent working on this book, they patiently (sometimes not so patiently) waited nearby, on my desk, in an adjoining chair, or just by my feet for a pet, pat, or snack.

# Preface

This is my personal story of learning to cope with Chronic Obstructive Pulmonary Disease (COPD). It is offered to you, not as a treatment handbook, but as a resource from a patient's perspective of the treatments available. The intention of writing this book is to simply share my experiences as a patient and what has "worked" for me. We are all very different and respond to treatment differently. It is my hope that this book will offer the reader an interesting balance of both a personal story as well as a useful resource of COPD treatment and rehabilitation information.

For the last ten years I have kept notes of my medical history and treatment. These notes were for my own personal reference to learn about my COPD. I often kept daily charts and records of my breathing capacity and medication doses. Later I made notes from the Pulmonary Rehabilitation classes, speakers, and COPD data from the Internet, COPD newsletters, and information from many discussions on COPD Lists. It was for my reference only and used often to prepare presentations when asked to speak to various groups.

References and quotes are noted in the paragraphs as they are used rather than in lengthy footnotes. My purpose is to give credit to the authors if known not to provide a scientific document or textbook.

When I decided to write a self-help book, I worried that I might not have unique information to share with my fellow lung patients. If my story is unique it is because I use the Mind-Body-

Spirit connection in managing my COPD. I have very severe emphysema and enjoy a fair amount of quality life. What I want most is to share what might work for you. If it is useful for you, I will be pleased with this opportunity to have helped. If it is not useful to you, pass it on to someone else who might learn from both of us.

Remember, we are not alone and always can learn from each other.

I have changed the names of fellow patients participating in treatment programs with me to protect their privacy. I have also changed the names of other medical professionals and any other identities of those I thought might prefer this privacy consideration. All other facts are authentic as they happen and to whom.

# Disclaimer:

*The purpose of this writing is to educate and entertain. The author shall have neither liability nor responsibility to any person or entity with respect to any loss or damage caused or alleged to have been caused, directly or indirectly, by the information contained in this book.*

*Before any changes are made in your particular medications or treatment regime, you must check with your physician. Your doctor must always know and approve of your treatment. He is your medical consultant.*

There are many other patients who have had different experiences and would welcome a debate on my perceptions. I admire their intellectual strengths but decline to debate the fact that we are different. If other challengers emerge for rightness or wrongness, I yield, they can be right.

I offer only love and understanding, empathy and compassion, for anyone's daily struggle with a chronic disability. No matter how bad my day gets, I always see someone in worse condition. I pray for them. I hope you will.

# Chapter 1

## The Beginning of Morbidity

In mourning who we once were . . . we must realize who we have become . . . and accept it. Coping with a chronic disability and coming to the realization that we will never be what we were, and even that we will never be able to enjoy the things that we once thought was the answer to happiness can be depressing. It does not have to be.

Morbidity is the rate of incidence of a disease, in my case, the advancing and debilitating effect of severe emphysema.

I will never forget the first time I was brought to my knees in the local emergency room with severe pneumonia. I had become very dehydrated, was running a high temperature, experienced severe difficulty of breathing and as I lay there on a gurney, I realized how frail, vulnerable, and very dependant I had become and how helpless I felt. The registered nurses and technicians were trying to start an intravenous tube, and just could not get the needle into a vein. They poked and poked first into my elbow area then into the top of my hands. It was painful as they dug around with a needle in my arm searching for my vein. Finally holding back the tears, begging them to find someone with better technique and skill, I hoped perhaps a lab technician or a doctor would try. Finally an anesthesiologist came to the emergency room and without further difficulty immediately started the intravenous (IV) flow of liquid in my vein. I was so grateful; never forgot him and years later thanked him at the medical center and told him how he was my angel that night.

I remember many years ago when I was a Navy Hospital Corpsman at Oak Knoll Hospital in Oakland, I made a promise to myself that if I ever tried to start an IV or draw blood, if I could not get the job done of getting the needle into a vein I would call someone else to do it. As the years would pass, I would experience this lack of skill many times. Laboratory technicians seem to be the most proficient at doing this job; may be because they do so many on a daily basis.

That night in the hospital emergency room was the first time that I would realize my life had changed. I must now learn to deal with the new fear of vulnerability; complete dependency. I would learn to yield and submit to the care or lack of it from others. It was the beginning of my realization that I would need to take control of managing my chronic obstructive pulmonary disease, commonly referred to as COPD.

*Chronic* simply means ongoing, not ending, pertaining to a condition that never goes away, does not get healed, or fixed in your body. *Obstructive* means obstructed, blocking, in my case, keeping air from moving in and out of my lungs. *Pulmonary* refers to lungs, the master organ of our body. The lungs supply all the other organs with oxygen through a very magnificent mechanism. Our lungs also balance the amount of oxygen and carbon dioxide in our blood. Our lungs are the only organs except the skin that expose themselves to the outside environment. Our lungs are exposed to contaminated air, toxins, smoke, dust, poison, virus, and other elements. Oh, yes, of course, to cigarette smoke. The word *disease* refers to a pathological condition.

COPD diagnosis normally includes Chronic Bronchitis, Asthma and Emphysema. Often the asthma component is removed from this COPD designation as many children suffer from asthma and sometimes outgrow this condition. One does not outgrow emphysema; as a matter of fact I am told that if one lives long enough, they will experience some emphysema.

Over sixteen million Americans today suffer from COPD, and

over 100,000 of them die each year. Most often emphysema is caused by cigarette smoke. I have spoken to hundreds of other patients about emphysema, in smoking cessation classes at our local medical center.

In trying to explain emphysema, I say that the tiny air sacs in the lower section of our lung lobes receive air filled with oxygen, process it by taking the oxygen from the air, filtering it through and into the blood giving off carbon dioxide to be exhaled back out of the lungs into the air.

This exhalation is aided by the contraction of the tiny air sacs called alveoli, much like a balloon deflating. Emphysema quite simply destroys this elasticity and these sacs become more like a paper bag, brittle, stiff, without any elasticity and thereby no longer contracts, helping the used air to leave our lungs.

As one can imagine, air becomes trapped in our diseased lungs taking up necessary space for new air, needed oxygen, and of course available space for our lungs to function. A pulmonary function test (PFT) measures the degree of impairment. The word emphysema comes from a Greek word *emphusema* meaning "inflation" and *emphusan* meaning "to blow in" . . . Actually emphysema more correctly impairs one's ability to "exhale," which of course takes up necessary space needed for newly inhaled air rich with oxygen.

My first smoking of cigarettes was by experimenting with smokes that I would steal from my father. Even before that, while my grandfather Arthur lived with us I became aware of cigar smoke. My very first recollections of him was in a cloud of blue smoke, puffing on a large King Edward cigar in his old stuffed chair behind a scowl and dirty eyeglasses. Usually shaking his head at the noise or a disagreement my older brother and sister and I were having.

Smoking was accepted in those days, the late 40's and early 50's—everyone seemed to smoke. Even before I thought it was cool, my neighbor and I would steal a cigar from my grandfather Arthur and hike to the family vegetable garden across the railroad tracks deep into the corn stalks and smoke. Choking and spitting,

I was only capable of handling a few drags and only enough to keep stride with my older brother often leaving the butt under a can for later retrieval.

I would often smell like smoke in school and be accused of smoking cigars. I hated the smell but everyone seemed to smoke everywhere in those days. I must have been twelve when I stepped up from cigars to cigarettes. Once I learned to tolerate a cigarette, the next thirty-five years of smoking would be history.

During the late 40's and early 50's, a pack of Lucky's or Camel's rolled up in my tee shirt sleeve was thought to be definitely cool.

As sometimes predicted medically, the first twenty years of smoking human lungs can somehow recover from cigarette smoke. At the twenty-year mark, things seem to change and continued smoking begins a series of bad consequences from lung cancer to high blood pressure, impotence, chronic bronchitis, chronic cough, and yes, emphysema. It was in fact after twenty years of smoking for me when my lung problems began.

I had finished my U.S. Navy tour of active duty as a Hospital Corpsman then spent a few years working with Hilton Hotels, which took me from Portland, Oregon, to New York, Chicago, and Beverly Hills, to the San Francisco Hilton Front Office. It was here, in 1965 that I met American airline pilots in flight training. It was twenty years after WW II. It seems post-war pilots were retiring in large numbers and pilot training programs to recruit new replacement pilots were available in every major airline.

I completed my Commercial Pilots Training, Flight Instructor, even Ground Instructor and Instrument Ratings just in time for hundreds of well-qualified pilots returning from Viet Nam looking for flying jobs. So, as it was, commercial airline pilot jobs were just not to be had by me at that time.

I returned to my home state Oregon and while flight instructing I learned about a flying job with the local sheriff's department. I remember the sheriff said to me, "Come to work and learn police work, when we get an airplane, you can fly it for us," "We have plans for an airplane in our budget." Well, I did and they didn't.

Twenty-five years later I was a retiring sheriff of the second largest county in Oregon, never having seen that promised airplane.

Smoking was easy in a job that never closed. Hospitals, hotels and sheriff departments never close; "Twenty-four seven," there was always something happening, always a shift to work, always cigarettes and coffee to consume.

In 1976, twenty years after I started smoking, while charging along in my Sheriff Department career, I seemed to have developed a nasty chronic cough. It was the first time, I heard the words from a doctor, *"You have some emphysema* on your chest x-ray and should stop smoking."

I told him I would try. I certainly did not "feel" any different, I did not hurt, could breathe as well as ever, so why quit? I didn't.

The next time I got a shocking reality check was five years later while in the Grand Cayman Islands, on my vacation with friends. We were looking forward to some pristine scuba and snorkel diving. My brother and I went to a swim dock to rent some scuba equipment. The qualification dive required us to put all the scuba gear on, descend to the bottom of the sea near the dock, about ten feet down, take all our gear off, lay it on the bottom then put it back on, clear the mask of water and return to the surface. We descended together, and proceeded to complete the test. I could not stay down and kept rising to the surface even with the weight belt. Air was trapped in my lungs, like built-in floats.

The dive shop operator required that we complete and sign a liability disclaimer form and one of the questions was regarding respiratory disease. I had to respond that I had been told that I had some emphysema. The large dark Cayman man, who appeared to be the shop operator, looked at me with his dark eyes and shook his head back and forth, "No way, my man, you can get narcosis." He explained further that I had air trapped in my lungs. I knew what he saying.

He and my brother assembled their scuba gear, dove into the clear aqua warm Caribbean waters and disappeared toward a shipwreck a few hundred yards off shore. I sat on the dock and had a cigarette while I waited.

On this trip, everyone had the scuba shipwreck experience except me. I sat on the beach smoking a cigarette and watched the bottom of the sea from the surface. I returned to Northwest Oregon where I continued to smoke two to three packs each day. This experience would stay with me for many years to come; it was the first life style change that I had to accept from my emphysema.

I did begin to focus on my breathing more; that is a bad sign of emphysema. Since I took my very first breath, breathing was an automatic response of my body. I was now noticing how and when I was getting air. I could not complete a yawn because of the shallow breath I noticed. Three flights of stairs in the old county courthouse where I worked every day would become too tough for me to climb. I would use the elevator, which for me was another life style change. When using the stairs, I was left without enough air to talk when I finally made it to the top floor.

By 1989, thirty-five years after my first cigarette, I frequently became conscious of my lack of air to breathe. I was smoking more and enjoying it less. I was finding fewer places that I could smoke. I was beginning to see that smoking was just not cool anymore. I had spent a lot of money on smoking cessation programs that failed for me. I would light up and decide that the program did not work and continued to smoke.

I was a 49-year-old divorced male. I very quickly realized that I was not very competitive in finding dates that included bike riding, skiing, walking, hiking, bowling, golfing, tennis, and even dancing. At one time I had enjoyed these things with the company of a woman. Another life style change was made without realizing it.

I met a lovely lady who had never smoked; she wanted to do some of these activities with me. It was humiliating for me to make excuses why I couldn't. I remember how difficult it was to find a place to smoke without offending her. I tried to keep the smell from my fingers, mustache and breath. After every cigarette I had a cleaning ritual, which became ridiculous. I would get ready for a date with her, get impatient waiting and light a cigarette, then wash my fingers, mustache, teeth, and begin waiting again, soon to become impatient and nervous, light a cigarette and start over again.

I had always loved to dance and country line dancing was new and a great place to meet other single people. I would wait on the sidelines until the song was almost over, then ask a lady to dance so I would not run out of air before the dance was over and still have air to talk to her.

This was the final warning for me; I knew, my life style was quickly changing and my activities of daily living had been compromised. It was the beginning of my disability. I knew I had to free myself of smoking. I wanted to be free from the smoke and death grip my lungs were suffering from. I knew what they must look like. I had seen autopsies in my work where the pathologist would say, "This is a smoker, see the dark tar-covered lung tissue"? I could not stand the thought of never smoking again. Cigarettes were my friends; they had been there whenever I needed a pause, a moment of reprieve to relax, a moment with my smoking friends, a social moment of relaxation and of acceptance. I did not know how not to smoke.

## Smoking Cessation

I finally decided I would not smoke cigarettes for one year. A thought that my mind could process and accept; I could always change my mind and start smoking at the end of a year. I had smoked for 35 years; I could at least give my lungs one year off from the toxic irritant. I told my girlfriend, Janet, whom I eventually married, that I would quit on New Year's Eve in 1989. I did and started the first minute of 1990, choosing not to smoke for one year. That evening I smoked and smoked until I ran out of time. I had three cigarettes left. We were at a New Year's Eve party at a friend's home and in front of everyone; I walked over to the fireplace and threw the remaining three cigarettes in the fire. Janet and I watched them burn. It was the beginning of a new life without cigarettes; little did I know how new and different it would be.

During the first week without cigarettes I had a chance to reflect on my life of smoking. I discovered I had all this extra time that I had used before to smoke. Just the fiddling with the pack, tapping the cigarette, lighting the end of it, watching it burn, flicking the ashes, walking over to the ashtray, finding a place to smoke, etc., lots of activity associated with smoking that takes time to do.

I also had a chance, now as a non-smoker, to reflect on the mind part of addiction, time to really remember, think about it, and understand why it had been so difficult to not smoke in the past.

Some of my memories were quite entertaining. I remembered on one of my birthdays that my former wife had given me a gift certificate for a session of acupuncture treatment to stop smoking. I was excited at the thought of this treatment and how I would walk away from it a non-smoker. Wow, how cool this could be, I thought as I drove to the clinic where the acupuncture was to be administered. When my turn came, I was escorted to the table where I lay still as the therapist carefully placed each needle in and around my ear.

After the treatment I walked to my car in the parking lot and while I started to drive away, I thought to myself, "I wonder if this treatment really worked"? This questioning thought only lasted a few moments before I said to myself, "There is only one way to know if it worked; Try it!" So I lit a cigarette and concluded, "Nope, it did not work," and smoked several cigarettes on the drive home. That evening, my wife said, "Well, honey, how did the treatment go?" I responded, "It didn't work" A similar scenario had also occurred with my hypnosis treatment. This time I made it to the bathroom to light up after the treatment to test the program's effectiveness. "It failed," I said to myself as I puffed on my cigarette.

I also tried two other smoking cessation programs, one that reduces the tar and nicotine in a strong cigarette to make it a weak one. Some of my thoughts are amusing; I recall rationalizing that with the reduced tar and nicotine it would be okay to smoke . . . but with the reduction I increased the amount of cigarettes I used each day to three packs.

With twenty cigarettes in each pack I smoked sixty cigarettes each day. Smoking three packs of cigarettes per day, sixty cigarettes, means that I must have smoked a cigarette every eighteen minutes if I was awake eighteen hours each day. Do the math: 18 hours x 60 minutes = 1080 minutes divided by 60 cigarettes = one every 18 minutes.

I had seen addiction of every kind in my work at the sheriff's department. I remember seeing the destruction of people's lives because of addictions. I had had long talks with inmates in our jail about all kinds of drug use. I had heard of inmates so desperately addicted to drugs that they would inject feces into their veins to get residual drugs. I was also familiar with alcohol addiction and the effect this "disease" had on crime of all kinds including domestic abuse and the involvement of children. I recalled the gambling addiction and conversations I have had with those who had "lost everything." I often wonder about the addiction of food and sex and how these devastating addictions adversely affect the quality of lives.

As I begin to understand my smoking addiction, I could easily see some similarities, and how our minds seem to be tricked into enabling the physical part of the addiction we may be feeding and how oblivious we become to how we yield to the addictions rather than learning to control them with our minds. I have studied the cognitive changes available to us in the way we perceive events and really began to see how thoughts control feelings which control our behavior. If I was able to change my thoughts then I knew I could change my smoking behavior.

I realized for the first time that to stop smoking I would have to change the way I recognized my feelings and thoughts about smoking. Wow! A breakthrough!

I made a promise that I have kept. I prayed for strength to stop smoking. I was willing to use all my resources this time. But I added a promise that if I was ever able to kick this smoking habit, if I could, that I would help others stop this debilitating habit. It has been twelve years since my last cigarette and I have spoken to hundreds of smokers while assisting at cessation classes.

There are volumes of writings on the subject of smoking cessation by many professionals who know more about human behavior than I do. One such person is Dr. James O. Prochaska at the University of Rhode Island who identified the "integrative model of change" and applied it to 872 people changing their smoking habits. The Prochaska five stages of change are: precontemplation, contemplation, action, maintenance, and release. This interesting information, as well as other helpful insights, can be found on the Internet. It is available to anyone interested in learning about our behaviors.

Because I promised that I would do what I could to help others stop smoking, I want to offer you some affirmations that helped me not to smoke that first year. If these are not particularly helpful to you, pass them on to someone else who is struggling with a smoking addiction.

## My "Non-Smoking" Affirmation List

I may always be a smoker, but I have chosen not to smoke now mainly because it is destroying my health and quality of life.

I have made the decision not to smoke. I do not "have to." I "get to" have this opportunity to control my life and what I do with my body.

I know and believe that I can choose not to smoke, live just fine, and actually be liberated from its control over my life.

I know I cannot trust my mind that may tell me that I "need" a cigarette, enabling me to continue this addiction that is trying to feed itself. The truth is, I *do not need* a cigarette. Not even one.

The "urges" to smoke will come whether I smoke or not: they will become less intense and less often as time passes. Urges are a sign of my healing from the smoking habit.

One cigarette is too many; three packs were not enough. If I smoke just one cigarette then I will have to "start over" withdrawing from this addiction. All my progress will be lost and my body will have new nicotine addiction to pass through again. My year of not smoking will start over.

As with any addiction, I must overcome my smoking one second at a time, then one minute, then one hour, one day, and then one week. The longer I go without a cigarette the less I will think I need one.

I know that living without breath is much worse than death. The important thing is how well I can live; and the quality of my next breath will determine that. I know that I cannot repair my lungs once they are damaged and that I can control what air or toxins I put into them. My lungs are exposed to my environment.

Smoking can also cause impotence in men; Not a good trade-off for smoking.

Everyone stops smoking, some die first! Think about it!

I can do it and I will keep my promise to help others stop smoking.

Note: I used to think I needed about twelve cigarettes every four hours . . . now I need a nebulizer breathing treatment every four hours. I spend over $1000 on medications per month just so I can breathe.

## An Earlier Promise

I remembered making a similar promise only once before. It was when I was a deputy sheriff. On a dark cold January morning in 1969 a deputy recruit named Bret and I were on the way to an injury accident. The roads were wet and we had a long way to go to get to the accident scene. As Bret drove the patrol vehicle through the winding roads of Oregon's rural western Washington county with lights flashing and siren wailing, I was watching the curves approach and disappear behind us. I reached down to tighten my seat belt and remembered that earlier that morning we learned that the passenger side seat belt would not fasten with the broken buckle. We tried to obtain another patrol car but one was just not available for us. In the final moments of navigating, as we turned onto the State Highway, we hit loose gravel, and the vehicle began spinning off of the roadway and rolled down an embankment. I saw the shotgun come loose from the dash holder, grabbed it to steady it while holding and bracing myself against the door with my right arm. Over and over we rolled. It was dark; the dirt and glass were everywhere, I could no longer tell which way was up or down or what direction the bouncing patrol car was going. Finally, on the last roll our car pitched up high, the passenger side down, I saw the ground coming up at me.

Then suddenly, the big cruiser stopped in midair, hung for just a moment, and rolled back down crashing to the ground, right side up. I could see daylight was dawning and could tell that we were in a field hundreds of yard from the roadway.

I had worked as a Navy Hospital Corpsman, in neurology and neurosurgery; I knew that I had broken my back or neck. When the police dispatcher finally determined where we were, the ambulance that had been sent to the accident that we were on our way to stopped to take me to the local hospital emergency room. Bret was okay except for a laceration on his nose.

I had seen my wife's pale face as she saw the cervical x-rays. Her name was Joan and she was one of the best emergency nurses

I have ever known. If her face was pale, I knew I was in trouble. I had been to surgery where they inserted tongs in my skull for cervical traction; as I lay in a striker frame on my back, I was told that I had fractured three vertebrae in my neck. The doctor told me that we would watch and wait and hope for the best, but I may have some paralysis from my chest down and that an iron lung was in the hallway "just in case" it was needed.

As I lay there flat on my back after taking some Demerol pain medication, with traction tongs in my skull, I wanted a cigarette. So I lit one up; yes, we could smoke in hospitals in those days; I became nauseated and wanted to vomit but could not turn my head to the side and this alarmed the nurses that I might be in trouble . . . I was.

The promise I made at that time to God was that I did not have the courage to be trapped in a dead body. I knew that I did not have what it takes to live that way. I promised God that if he would spare me this one time that I would never complain again about anything. I further promised that I would develop my mind, so if necessary I would not need to exclusively depend on my physical body. God does keep his promises, and one week later I left the hospital in a four-post neck brace that I lived in for the next three months.

I returned to work at the sheriff's department where I was able to sit on a swivel chair and dispatch while on light duty. I was finally released to full duty a year later. I learned that one's life could change in an instant. I eventually returned to my complaining and felt guilty about the promise. Fourteen years later I was elected sheriff.

# Chapter 2

## Chronic Obstructive Pulmonary Disease (COPD)

Many COPD studies continue to be conducted; the most recent at the time of this writing offers an excellent overview of how we currently see or do not see this disease.

### *Tuesday, October 2, LONDON (Reuters)*

"People suffering from lung diseases often do not receive the right treatment because they do not know what they are suffering from or how serious it is."

The first international survey of chronic obstructive pulmonary disease, or COPD, which includes emphysema and chronic bronchitis, showed that 20% of people with the illness could not name it and 46% continued to smoke, even though smoking is the leading cause of the disease. Patients also underestimated the seriousness of their illness, according to the survey reported in the *European Respiratory Journal (ERJ)* on Tuesday, October 2, 2002.

"The data published in the present issue of the *ERJ* suggest that despite their complaints and the significant limitations in their daily life activities, COPD sufferers underestimate their morbidity (quality of life) and their disorder is undertreated,"

Professor Richard Dekhuijzen, of the University Medical Center in Nijmegen in the Netherlands, as quoted in an editorial.

In the poll conducted by Stephen Rennard of the University of Nebraska Medical Center in Omaha and colleagues in Canada and Europe, patients who admitted they had to stop walking even at a moderate pace described their illness as mild. Many sufferers who said they walked slower than most people of their age also thought their condition was not serious.

According to the survey, 64% of patients were treated by their general practitioners and only 20% had been examined by a respiratory specialist.

Rennard and his colleagues said only 45% of patients had had a detailed lung function test and 39% received no medication for their illness.

COPD, which affects more than 16 million people in the U.S. alone, causes progressive damage to the lungs. Shortness of breath, chronic and mild cough and fatigue are symptoms of the illness also. Dekhuijzen said important lessons can be learned from the survey, which was conducted in the United States, Canada, France, Italy, Spain, the Netherlands, Germany and Britain.

Firstly, patients need to be made aware of the severity of the disease.

Secondly, the disease must be given a label: "It is not normal that only 20% of patients should be aware that they suffer from COPD," he explained.

People should become familiar with COPD because it is a severe and disabling illness, he added.

I tried to recall the first time a doctor told me that I had COPD. It seems it was during one of my bouts with a chronic cough that lingered for months during and after a common cold. I recall he said something about chronic bronchitis and gave me my first medication inhaler. Metered dose inhalers are the "puffers" you see patients using. It is a canister under pressure of a propellant with a specified amount of medication measured in grams and dispensed one puff at a time. The most common are the ones prescribed containing a bronchodilator to expand the airways to our lungs. This was my first. I did not know much about the medication; its side effects, proper use, spacers, or proper cleaning methods which were not explained to me. I had used one for years before learning this information. I meet COPD patients frequently that have never cleaned their inhalers or spacers. The inhalers cost approximately $50 each and like all medications, the cost keeps increasing.

The first mention of COPD and the beginning use of inhaled medication were so quickly accepted that I thought nothing of it. My doctor and I were smoking at that time and it seemed to never be a major health issue that we discussed. It was a common sight to see me inhale medication so I could open my airways and stop coughing just to facilitate the smoking of a cigarette.

I read about a lung study in our local newspaper being conducted at our university hospital by a pulmonologist, who was apparently evaluating Alpha 1 Antitrypsin Deficiency in a study group. The American Lung Association defines Alpha 1 as follows:

"Alpha-1 related emphysema or Alpha-1 deficiency is caused by an inherited lack of a protective protein called alpha-1 antitrypsin (AAT). In normal and healthy individuals, AAT protects the lungs from a natural enzyme (called neutrophil elastase) that helps fight bacteria and cleans up dead lung tissue. However, this enzyme can also eventually damage lung tissue if not neutralized by AAT. If allowed to progress, this form of emphysema becomes chronic and lung tissue continues to be destroyed; eventually it is fatal if the progress is not slowed down or halted. Every person inherits two AAT genes, one from each parent. A person has AAT Deficiency (Alpha-1) only if he or she inherits two abnormal genes.

People who have only one abnormal gene and one normal AAT gene are "carriers" Their AAT levels may be lower than normal, but not as low as the deficiency state, and their risk of significant health problems is much lower than those with the severe deficiency.

People who have Alpha-1 deficiency will pass on one abnormal gene to their children. They will be "carriers" and will not have Alpha-1 unless they receive an abnormal gene from their other parent. There are tests for determining if a person is a carrier or is AAT deficient. These tests are called genotyping and phenotyping.

It was my very first introduction to a pulmonary function test (PFT). I would come to experience these test many times over the next ten years.

*The Gale Encyclopedia of Medicine* defines PFT as follows:

> "Pulmonary function tests are a group of procedures that measure the function of the lungs, revealing problems in the way a patient breathes. The tests can determine the cause of shortness of breath and may help confirm lung diseases, such as asthma, bronchitis or emphysema. The tests also are performed before any major lung surgery to make sure the person won't be disabled by having a reduced lung capacity.
>
> Pulmonary function tests can help a doctor diagnose a range of respiratory diseases which might not otherwise be obvious to the doctor or the patient.
>
> The tests are important since many kinds of lung problems can be successfully treated if detected early. The tests are also used to measure how a lung disease is progressing, and how serious the lung disease has become.
>
> Pulmonary function tests also can be used to assess how a patient is responding to different treatments.
>
> One of the most common of the pulmonary function tests is *spirometry* (from the Greco-Latin term, meaning "to measure breathing"). This test, which can be given in a hospital or in a doctor's office, measures how much and how fast the air is moving in and out of the lungs. Specific measurements taken during the test include the volume of air from start to finish, the fastest flow that

is achieved, and the volume of air exhaled in the first second of the test.

A peak flow meter can determine how much a patient's airways have narrowed.

A test of blood gases is a measurement of the concentration of oxygen and carbon dioxide in the blood, which shows how efficient the gas exchange is in the lungs. Another lung function test reveals how efficient the lungs are in absorbing gas from the blood. This is measured by testing the volume of carbon monoxide a person breathes out after a known volume of the gas has been inhaled.

When I checked in at the university hospital for my first PFT "test" I knew something had changed drastically in my lungs. I had learned to avoid stairs or inclines because I was experiencing shortness of breathe ( SOB), medically referred to as "dyspnea," meaning difficulty breathing. Unless one has experienced an alarming shortness of breath they cannot possibly understand how frightening it can be. I once thought I would suffocate when I experienced this terror. I cope with it now, almost daily, but never really get comfortable when it happens. People with COPD and especially emphysema must relearn how to breathe and actually control the panic of feeling as if they are about to suffocate. *When one cannot breathe, nothing else matters.*

It was one of my bad breathing days when I went for this first test. I had difficulty finding a parking place anywhere near the entrance; the parking structure was full, and there were no elevators. I struggled across the lot, resting every ten steps or so. I then climbed the wheelchair ramp as if it were a mountain. Each step, one slowly in front of the next; it was exhausting. Finally entering the lower hall, I was confused regarding which direction to go. I would also much later learn confusion is a symptom of lack of oxygen in our blood. Panic and confusion feeds itself with fear. Many years later I would be teaching this self-perpetuated anxiety as the "fear dyspnea cycle."

Finding an elevator, I made it to the upper floor where the respiratory department was located. It seems so simple to me that to make access easier for emphysema patients, the respiratory department should be located on the bottom floor of a clinic instead on the upper floor. I entered a dimly lit room full of computers and tubes. A very friendly respiratory therapist greeted me and explained the details of the test. He commented that a clip would be placed on my nose; deep breathing in and especially out, emptying my lungs would be measured on the computer. He began with a chest x-ray, commenting to me I will need to take it again. "I missed the lower part of your lungs." I learned months later that this condition of expanded lungs is "hyperinflation." It is common among emphysema patients. The lungs "over inflate" into the lower cavity of the chest requiring a longer x-ray photo to include the desired chest area for x-ray. This hyperinflated expansion of one's lungs in an effort to compensate for the damaged tissue dysfunction of the lower lobes is a common complication of emphysema.

In the years that followed, I learned to tell x-ray technicians that my lungs had hyperinflated deep into my thoracic cavity against my diaphragmatic breathing muscle and to my belt line.

The large dark male respiratory therapist seemed kind and gentle as he explained each of the pulmonary function tests. Over and over again I would take a deep breath then exhale longer and longer as I thought my head and red bulging face would burst. With my red face and veins distended, I would push trapped air from my lungs and watch the needle on the computer graph paper move slowly, making a record of my lung capacity.

The therapist would often do retesting including recalibrating the test equipment. He gave me an inhaler for medication; we waited ten minutes then began the testing over again. At the conclusion of the test, I asked him, "How did I do?" He replied, "Doctor will review the results with you. We are done with this part; we will now go to the lab to take a blood sample."

I had only a brief conversation with the pulmonologist that day, who told me that I had some advanced emphysema, probably from smoking, and prescribed some additional medications. I asked him about the prognosis and potential treatment of my COPD disease. He seemed evasive in saying it was "hard to tell, everyone is different."

I left the hospital and struggled to get back up the steep parking lot to find my car. Weeks later I received a letter from the Registry of Patients with Deficiency of Alpha 1-Antitrypsin, which informed me the pulmonary tests had revealed that, "You have intermediate deficiency, most of your obstructive lung disease is due to your past history of cigarette smoking." I later learned that I was not a good candidate for the study. This was eleven years ago and seems like a lifetime.

## A Change in Life Style

The year 1993 was a very different year for me. It was full of tragedy and loss that I somehow needed to find a way to cope. I was winding down a twenty-five-year career, decided not to run for the office of sheriff and planned to retire.

I was short six months from the end of my term as elected sheriff for the twenty-fifth anniversary of my employment in our retirement system. I needed somehow to bridge this gap if possible. I had announced that I was not going to run the year before and became a public office "lame duck." A lame duck is an elected official that is finishing his or her term of office after they have publicly announced they are *not* going to seek reelection. I had indeed been a politically neutered lame duck.

I had watched my predecessor and other sheriffs run and be elected to office then retire a few months later. Thinking it would be better for the people I served, I carefully prepared a replacement, endorsed him, worked on his campaign and after his election I became a target for anyone who felt they needed retribution from previous disagreements with me. I learned why other elected officials leave public office while elected. I witnessed my replacement avoid this situation, ten years later, by getting reelected then retiring. He had learned from my mistake, enjoyed his power right up to the day he left office. This is an interesting lesson in politics for any student of strategy willing to learn this political reality.

That same year, my father died of a heart attack, and considering how dependent my mother had become on him, I wondered how she might survive being alone. They had been married over fifty years and they were dependent upon each other.

I had struggled through a very sad divorce in 1990, lost my financial base and was emotionally drained from the experience. I had been introduced to "depression" and how it can distort life's events to the point of complete unhappiness. I was really feeling like I was at the bottom of a pit.

Finally in 1993, I was forced to meet head-on my decreasing physical ability with diseased lungs. I had stopped smoking three years earlier and was still waiting to recover . . . it just did not happen. I never regained my lung function and started to realize how badly they had been damaged from thirty-five years of cigarette smoking.

I was a mess and had to make a change if I were to get through it. "I needed to get out to get up," if you know what I mean. The brightest things in my life and certainly the most helpful at the time were my friends Janet, Erica, and two male Siamese guys. My cat guys were giving me a reason to get up in the morning. I wondered who would take care of these little blue-eyed fur balls if something happened to me. I had to find a slower way of living and a more peaceful place. I decided that at the end of the year, I would return to my hometown on the Northwestern Oregon Columbia River Gorge. To a rural Oregon town of 12,000 people offering 300 days of blue sky and sunshine with less than ten inches of rain per year. Who knows, I thought, I could even be some help to my mom.

It was an interesting experience for me to live with my mom for a few weeks until I could find a house to buy. I realized I had never gotten to know her as an adult. My annual visits had been limited to holidays and as the years past I never realized that I had not taken the time as an adult to know her. She never stopped relating to me as one of her kids, and for some reason she was unable to accept that I was an older adult.

I was spending the weekends one hundred miles away in Lake Oswego with my Janet and Siamese guys. I then returned to the Gorge during the week while I searched for a home to buy. This life style was scattered and unsettling and actually added to the stress I had brought with me.

I began to volunteer at the local medical center in their transportation program, driving patients to medical appointments. There were a dozen or so of us, older retired drivers who volunteered to take mostly patients in "wheelchair lift"-equipped vans to doctor's appointments and medical treatments. It was a great service; there was no available bus or taxi service in the city, we were "it" for many older people. The medical center provided this service free to the residents in our area . . . an unbelievably successful program.

Although this program was later incorporated with other volunteer driver programs and transferred to a public transportation system where it appropriately belonged, it was a great introduction to volunteer work for me. I became familiar with the medical center and its personnel.

My health continued to deteriorate. Progressing slowly each day, I began to learn how to compensate by hiding my disability. I knew I could no longer keep up. Janet and I stopped going to smoky country-dance clubs that we were accustomed to.

I found and purchased a little 1200-square-foot ranch-style, single-level double-garage home. I quickly learned my breathing difficulty was keeping me from doing yard work and finally found neighborhood kids to mow my lawn. I could not walk to the mailbox, could not walk through a grocery or variety store without sitting down. I had trouble finishing a shower without resting. I could no longer get dressed without resting after each item of clothing was put on. I was continuing to gain weight from the corticosteroid medication I was taking. I began to limit myself to the volunteer office, staying indoors to avoid more activity and the cold air that I simply could not breathe.

While at home I began to find myself out in the yard trying to work. More and more I was dealing with the panic of suffocation, thinking I could not get to the house or to a phone for needed help if necessary. I found I would have to sit on the ground until I calmed myself. I would often rush to find my recovery medication inhaler and then not have enough air left to inhale the medication. I just knew I would soon die of suffocation.

I continued to see my doctor in Portland and learned of a new lung treatment procedure called lung volume reduction surgery (LVRS). About the same time, Frances, one of the dear ladies in the volunteer office, asked me if I had ever applied for Social Security Disability (SSD). Both of these bits of news gave me hope and a realization that I must learn more about my disease. I knew that I must take charge of my own destiny. I was headed for the bottom "quality of life" in just doing the activities of daily living (ADLs).

By then, I had gained fifty pounds, most of which parked on my abdomen, increasing my waist size by eight inches. I was miserable, sick, depressed, and ready for some new hope, new leads, and hungry for knowledge that I badly needed to survive.

## I Am Not Alone

One day, while volunteering in the office at the medical center, I learned that a new pulmonary support group called "Better Breathers" was being organized and I was invited to attend. This was the beginning of my rehabilitation and education. The American Lung Association and our state chapter coordinate local clubs to support Better Breather's Clubs. This was in late September of 1996. Our State American Lung Association describes the Better Breather's Club as follows:

The American Lung Association of Oregon (ALAO) has many resources on preventing and living with Chronic Obstructive

Pulmonary Disease (COPD). ALAO also supports Better Breathers Clubs for patients, family members, friends, or anyone interested in the better management of COPD. The Better Breathers Club (BBC) combines educational information with informal sharing and social opportunities. These educational programs include videos, literature demonstrations and presentations by guest physicians, respiratory therapists and other healthcare and social welfare professionals.

The "Better Breather Clubs" includes people helping people—an opportunity for mutual support and sharing ideas and experiences. BBC groups usually meet on a monthly basis in locations throughout the state. Joining a group is a simple matter of contacting the American Lung Association and calling the coordinator for the group nearest you.

I entered the small meeting room at our local medical center that day of my first meeting with the "Better Breathers Club" with my lovely wife, Janet. My observation was that everyone seemed older than I was by at least ten years. Some were using oxygen from a portable green tank with a regulator and tube running into their noses. The hissing sound of their breathing was at first alarming. The meeting facilitator was a short attractive woman who seemed warm and friendly. She was introduced as the medical center director of respiratory therapy.

I kept Janet at my elbow, as always when I was in a new situation, to talk for me if I ran out of breath and could not communicate. I was winded from the walk to the medical center from the parking lot. Locating the meeting room had taken extra steps and air that I did not have.

It is impossible to explain to someone who has not experienced it what it is like to depend on another to speak for him or her. Since we all think and speak differently using the expressions and vocabulary we know . . . no one else can articulate what we want and how we want it said like we can.

I was learning to depend on Janet to speak for me and it was difficult for both of us. As hard as she tried to please me, her comments were either late, slow, or not exactly what I would have said and she would be the recipient of my "laser look" and me of hers. I am sure it is as piercing as any arrow directly into her heart. I have never been able to get used to this part of my disability. I can now understand how those who cannot speak must feel. It is humbling. Usually by the time we got it straight on what I wanted her to say, I would impatiently begin to blurt out short statements, as I was able to blurt out air and talk, always feeling like I sounded like a fool.

I always wanted to speak softly and quietly, slow and strong, unobtrusive and more articulate. When I am out of air, I know I sound exactly the opposite with my loud burst of air. My voice and air volume are without quality and I am unable to hide my emotions and breathing problem. This condition does cause stress and embarrassment causing a normal voice to change quality.

Two very useful pieces of information came from that first meeting of Better Breathers. First and most powerful was the realization that "*I was not alone,*" that there were other people coping with the struggle for the same lung disease that I had. They seemed to have the same feelings and needs as I had.

I noticed a lack of knowledge and understanding about our disease in some of the other patients. Most, if any, did not have computers and had not had the opportunity to visit the world of information on the cyberspace super highway. I had just purchased my first computer and began to surf for information on lung disease. Some new "Lung Lists" of people with lung problems were just forming and I had begun learning from others with COPD, Alpha 1, sarcoidosis and other diseases from all over the country and abroad. It is an amazing resource and a further confirmation that I was not alone in my struggle. I could learn a lot from others . . . I would ask questions.

# Chapter 3

## Rehabilitation Ready

The second and most exciting piece of information I learned from my first Better Breathing club meeting was the medical center was starting the first class offered for pulmonary rehabilitation. We were invited to apply with a required doctor's prescription order for this program as well as a breathing pre-rehabilitation assessment.

The Cheshire Medical Center, Dartmouth explains the Pulmonary Rehabilitation Program as follows: The pulmonary rehabilitation program at the Cheshire Medical Center is designed for patients with chronic respiratory disease (COPD, emphysema, chronic bronchitis, pulmonary fibrosis, and other conditions). The program combines education with therapeutic exercise and functional activities into a comprehensive twelve-week program. The goal is to help the patient understand and cope with the disease and function more comfortably and independently at home.

With a doctor's referral, the program coordinator will conduct an evaluation. If you are found to be appropriate for admission to the program, a team of healthcare professionals will evaluate your current level of functioning. An individualized program to meet your needs will be designed just for you. Your pre-program evaluation will include full pulmonary function studies, laboratory tests, EKG and a cardiac stress test as well as a consultation with a physician who specializes in pulmonary medicine.

## Summary of A Rehabilitation Program

The first session begins with an orientation to your program.
Some activities will take place individually and others with a group of patients dealing with similar breathing problems. You will come to the program two days each week. Your visits will last approximately three hours and you will be given an exercise plan to continue at home at least one to two additional times per week. Your exercise program will begin at a level based on your ability. It will start slowly and progress toward your goal each week.

Educational lectures and activities will cover a wide range of topics designed to help you fully understand your disease and give you the information you need to improve function and feel better. During the regular support groups you will have the opportunity to share your questions and concerns with others dealing with similar challenges. Your progress will be continually monitored and adjustments will be made to your program based on your individual performance.

The goal, it seems, is to provide you with the skills and knowledge necessary to *improve your quality of life while dealing with a chronic breathing disability*.

Our local program, which started for the first time in late November 1996, began with approximately six COPD patients. The newly constructed facility called "Center for Mind Body Medicine" at our medical center, also known as a Plaintree Facility. Our pulmonary rehabilitation program became one of the first such programs in our area. We started our program with a nine-week curriculum, including the following topics:

Breathing Techniques
Exercise with Limited Capabilities
Medication Management

Respiratory Concepts
Nutrition & Weight Management
Stress Reduction and Relaxation Techniques
Travel & Leisure Planning with COPD

Because my lung disease had reduced me to "disabled" and the quality of my  life had deteriorated . . . I had become very receptive and motivated  to participate in this program.

Two other events in 1996 confirmed my level of disability and had robbed  me of any hope of ever getting "well" or even better. In late 1995, two years after I retired and my life became one of coping with shortness of breath and a daily battle against suffocation, my physician, a very dear woman that had cared for me in the most compassionate way ever, referred me to Oregon Pulmonary Associates for a pulmonary consultation.

This consultation requested many tests including the pulmonary function tests, CT lung scans, high-density lung x-rays, a nuclear lung scan as well as a thoracic surgical consultation. One of the purposes of these consultations was to determine if I was a suitable candidate for lung volume reduction surgery (LVRS) or a lung transplant (TX). It had been a stressful week for Janet and me, including the four-hour round trip drive through the winter conditions of the Columbia River Gorge to the large medical facility in Portland for these tests.

It was an overcast, gray, cold afternoon following the nuclear lung scan that we finally got the results of most of the PFT testing and the results of the x-rays.

The thoracic surgeon was a big man, well groomed, and kind, who spoke in a gentle but very firm way. He was dressed in green surgical scrubs with a white coat, untied mask and surgical cap. I noted from his nametag that his first name was "Storm." I thought to myself it was ironic and was amused for a moment, Now how could I possibly get good news from a man who was named "Storm"?

I am sure I had often appeared flip trying to hide my fear of the inevitable unknown. Storm was very kind to us; he explained that my tests revealed severe advanced emphysema with a diffusion impairment. He explained further that I was not a very good candidate for thoracic surgery. I did not have a good lung or part of lung that would get me through chest surgery. He said that he would "not open a man's chest if he could not make him better." I asked him what I always end up asking doctors when I had discussed treatment; it is the only thing I know how to ask, "What would you do if you had these lungs?" He replied, "I would not have surgery now, I would make treatment plans and wait until I had no other options."

Janet and I sat in the waiting room, near x-ray; she began to cry and asked me, "What now, what would be next?" I replied, "We will take one day at a time, that is all we ever get." The next day I recall getting a call from a friend of mine in the metropolitan area asking about my lungs for they had heard that I was getting a lung transplant. I wondered how private news traveled so fast in such a large city. I had forgotten that I was well known from being the sheriff in the county where this hospital was located and it apparently seems newsworthy to someone.

In February 1996 my doctor received the results of this evaluation. This letter addressed to my primary care physician, from the Pulmonary Associates, which was sent to the Review Department, Health Plan to request approval for insured treatment of LVRS. The written request was a requirement to see if further treatment would be covered by my insurance. I have learned that one's insurance company . . . and *not* the physician requesting the needed treatment most often decides one's treatment. I seem to observe the "tail is wagging the dog" in deciding our available medical care in America.

## A letter from my pulmonologist reads as follows:

*I write regarding Mr. Probstfield, your insured. He has severe advanced emphysema with an FEV 1 of 0.6 liters, a diffusion impairment, and little response to bronchodilators. His exercise status is severely compromised and he finds that he is able to do very little for himself in the way of exertion.*

*Over the past several months, attempts were made to manage him medically.*

*However, there has been no substantial change in his condition with the institution of the various medications available in the therapeutic armamentarium for emphysema. For this reason, he has been considering both lung transplantation and, as a bridge to this procedure, lung reduction surgery. A significant amount of workup has been undertaken for this purpose, as you will see from examining his records.*

*The purpose of this communication is to officially request authorization for evaluation at Oregon Health Sciences University for lung transplantation. I would like to get him going on this track in the very near future. In addition, I would like to request authorization for a lung reduction surgery procedure, which would be performed in the near future as a bridge towards transplantation.*

*The list for patients with emphysema is exceedingly long and Mr. Probstfield probably cannot count on a transplant within two years.*

*I will wait to hear from you further regarding this request.*

*Sincerely, (My Pulmonologist)*

The American Lung Association simply describes Lung Volume Reduction Surgery as follows: "Lung volume reduction surgery is a surgical procedure in which the most severely diseased portions of the lung are removed to allow the remaining lung and breathing muscles to work better. The short term results are promising but those with severe forms are at higher risk of death."

Timing is everything and often determines if opportunities can happen. It might have been a twist of fate or just coincidence in late 1996, about the same time I was seeking this LVRS treatment, thinking that I only had five years left of any life quality.

For example, I had a friend I knew from high school who became a firefighter. He was a heavy cigarette smoker, diagnosed with emphysema about the same time I was, qualified for a lung transplant, got on a waiting list for a donor organ and died while waiting for the "call" to have it done. Jim became what I did not want to have happen to me. He spent the last few years of his life in an easy chair with a TV remote control as his companion while sucking on a tube from a green oxygen bottle; not for me, I thought.

Anyway, timing is critical and by late 1996 . . . and about the time many emphysema patients were clamoring to get the lung volume reduction surgery that was appearing in the national news, Medicare decided to stop paying for it. Since there seemed to be ambiguity in protocol and procedure and a lack of standardization among the surgeons performing this surgery it was quickly classified as "experimental" rendering it non-authorized for payment by Medicare.

The National Heart, Lung and Blood Institute (NHLBI) and the Health Care Financing Administration (HCFA), including the National Institute of Health, the federal government's health research agency (NIH), are the government agencies that oversee Medicare approved treatment. This group of distinguished professionals decided to do a clinical trial to compare the benefits and risks of two or more methods of treatment.

This trial was named National Emphysema Treatment Trial (NETT) and seventeen participating medical centers were selected. They were University of Michigan in Ann Arbor, University of Maryland John Hopkins Hospital in Baltimore, Brigham and Women's Hospital in Boston, Cleveland Clinic in Cleveland, Ohio State University in Columbus, National Jewish Center U of Colorado in Denver, Duke University in Durham, Baylor College of Medicine in Houston, Cedars-Sinai Medical Center in Los Angeles, Long Island Jewish Medical Center in New Hyde Park NY, Columbia University in NY, Temple University in Philadelphia, University of Pittsburgh in Pittsburgh, Mayo Clinic in Rochester, University of California in San Diego, University of Washington in Seattle, and St. Louis University in St. Louis, Missouri.

This research study was to compare lung volume reduction surgery to other treatments for emphysema. The "other" treatment was often called "medical" and the LVRS was called "surgical." Both pre and post NETT participating patients were required to complete extensive and standardized pulmonary rehabilitation programs to either measure the results of treatment or prepare for the surgical procedure.

The interesting fact was that the patients did not know which treatment they would receive, medical or surgical, and could not choose when entering the program. So a patient like me who had completed medical rehabilitation and wanted to get the surgery may end up just doing the pulmonary rehab program which some had already done. A 50% random selection was made to determine who got what treatment program. I believe this put a damper on willing NETT study participants. The program was substantially delayed in getting started. The methodology of surgical procedure was difficult to get all seventeen medical centers to agree on, and finally some patients began to mortgage their homes or get loans and fund their own $30,000 to $50,000 surgery.

Medicare stopped all approval for this surgery until the NETT study was completed and the effectiveness of this surgery was determined and published.

What this NETT study meant to me and to thousands of other emphysema patients was simply that this surgical procedure, LVRS, would not be available to us for three to five years. This procedure appeared to be the only surgical treatment that existed at the time to relieve the terrible obstructive symptoms of shortness of breath we all had to live with daily. The closest participating medical center for me was Seattle, Washington. I would need to move my residence to Seattle for several months to even consider this option. We learned that after transplantation and sometimes with LVRS, the post-surgical routine is very intrusive in one's life with major life style changes.

Postoperative pulmonary patients have often been on high doses of antibiotics, anti-rejection medications, corticosteroids, weekly blood draws, intrusive exams, and biopsies. Their compromised immune system becomes more compromised and they are more susceptible to respiratory infections. It can be a very tough rehabilitation period for some patients. I have been told that in the last few years this post-surgical treatment has become less intrusive.

We decided that we would wait; Medicare, our group or supplemental insurance would not pay. One medical insurance processing clerk finally admitted to me that my medical insurance company had stated: "You seem to be doing too well now for transplantation and we are not doing LVRS," a very diplomatic way of saying, "Too bad for you, we are not paying." Translated to us it meant there was no treatment to fix my broken lungs.

The good thing regarding this unavailable surgery is that many patients who thought this surgery was a cure were not good candidates for this treatment. It delayed further mistakes of people having it and suffering bad results. It forced many to consider the "medical" treatment of pulmonary rehabilitation. At the time of this writing some preliminary findings have been published by the NETT. Although some participating patients realized immediate results, the improvement did not last beyond three years; for others it was shorter. Some patients did not survive the surgical experience beyond thirty days; others are on their third to fifth year of improvement. As a result people with severe emphysema will no longer be admitted to the NETT study.

Between three and five years postoperative improvement seems to depend on continued rehabilitation efforts, diet, exercise, medication management, and many other factors. Many of the factors necessary to maintain maximum lung capacity are the same factors necessary for non-postoperative patients. Thus the "medical model" seems to provide many of the same long-term benefits without surgery. Today, I am grateful we decided (with the influence of the NETT circumstances) to avoid major surgery on my lungs at the time we were considering it. Storm was correct in his advice to us. We will always be grateful to him.

## Social Security Disability

The next event that confirmed my disability was applying for Social Security Disability. From the day that wonderful caring lady in the volunteer office of the medical center suggested I apply, I have heard horror stories of difficulty and rejection. From the moment that I applied at our local Social Security Office I was assisted in every way through the application process. I took the application packet home and completed all the blanks. In the application packet I included my three rejection letters refusing me life insurance, the pulmonary function test results and the letter from my pulmonologist requesting insurance approval for a lung transplant. I also included a description of my difficulty with doing some activities of daily living (ADL) and submitted the packet to Social Security.

Within a few weeks my request was approved including two years of back payment. This unexpected Social Security Disability assistance has been a great help to me. A wonderful bonus to this approval in qualifying for SSD is being qualified to receive Medicare. For me it was at age 55 instead of waiting until I was 65. I am eternally grateful for this help. I worked all my life and have maximum work credits to draw upon. It saved any possible quality of life for me being unable to do meaningful work. I am sad some other COPD patients do not seem to be able to access this assistance. I avoid judgment because I have seen so many different cases and denial reasons for Social Security of these disability claims. My disability was confirmed to me by their approval of my claim; it was no longer subjective. My disabled condition was now a matter of medical record . . . evaluated and documented.

It was time for me to get to work in managing my health, my life, and my destiny.

I am not a physician, pharmacist, caregiver or healthcare professional. I am a COPD patient who has struggled and learned to manage his disability. The pulmonary rehabilitation experience that I am about to share with you will help *if* you commit yourself in a determined way to learn what you can from me as well as others who will share their experiences. We can learn much from each other which people who do not live with COPD cannot relate to.

Like I wrote earlier, I gained over fifty pounds and nine inches on my waist during the last few years before I enrolled in pulmonary rehabilitation. This is a common side effect from corticosteroids, tablets or inhaled. I had also developed the beginning of panic attacks from fear of suffocating. It was November 1996, I was ready for pulmonary rehabilitation; it was the only game in town—win, lose or draw, sink or swim, fish or cut bait, I had absolutely nothing to lose. I needed help or I knew I would be spending my time in a recliner with a television remote control, watching my life go by without me.

# Chapter 4

## Pulmonary Rehabilitation—
## The Body

My pulmonary rehabilitation experience started the moment I reported to Diane, the respiratory therapist and director of this new program named pulmonary rehabilitation. I was skeptical. Diane is an attractive, well-dressed woman with a beautiful smile. A young professional, fit, and energetic physical therapist named Wanda joined her as staff in the program. They both were really interested and excited about this opportunity to work with pulmonary patients in this new way.

The rehabilitation was to be conducted in a new Pulmonary Health and Rehabilitation Program. As a result of a conflict with other established programs, the name was eventually changed to "Center for Mind Body Medicine" and Pulmonary and Cardiac Rehabilitation.

It was in November when we started this class and the weather had begun to get colder in Northwest Oregon. Cold air is very difficult to breathe with emphysema. My wife Janet and I arrived for the pre-screening early. Janet knows me to have a "Type-A" personality and I seem to fuss and push to always be early for appointments even if it does not matter.

I had learned to always give myself extra time. I usually needed this time to get dressed, remember to take my medications and my walk to the car, etc.

I had become accustomed to this extra slow movement and leaving myself extra time for my needed routine. I would sit on the bed, put one foot in one trouser leg, then rest to get my breath. Put the other leg in a trouser and rest. Put one arm in my shirt and rest to get more air. Put the other arm in the other shirt sleeve and rest. Walk a few steps and rest to get more air. Put one shoe on and rest. Put the other shoe on and rest. It was the same that November day in the parking lot at pulmonary rehabilitation. I would walk a few steps and rest, taking extra time to get to the classroom.

Upon entering this new facility we felt as though we were at an expensive health club. The beautifully carpeted and decorated room resembled a fitness center. I was overweight, huffing and puffing and without enough air to do the normal greeting and other talking that I wanted to. Everyone seemed to understand. I quickly found my most direct route to a chair and sat down grabbing for my Albuterol inhaler and took a couple of quick puffs. There were five of us in this class, the rest were older than I was, but other than that they were struggling to breathe as I was. The three male student patients were accompanied by assisting spouses. The other two were women and alone.

I have come to realize how fortunate anyone is who copes with a disability in having a partner that will help you through it. It takes such courage and effort to do it alone. I admire the men and women I have seen cope with COPD on their own without the assistance of a spouse or significant other.

Janet did stay by my side that day. We all completed a physical assessment to determine a pre-rehab level of fitness, activity capabilities, and the degree of our lung dysfunction. Some measures of fitness included a six-minute walk, treadmill, upper body exerciser, stationary bike, and a combination of arm and leg machine exercise. Some hand weights and stretch bands are also used.

Oxygen levels are measured by a finger devise called an oximeter. Vital signs: blood pressure, pulse and respiration are taken before and after each rehab session. The subjective level of perceived breathlessness by the patient is also recorded. This measurement is usually determined on a scale from 1, indicating a very slight feeling of breathlessness, to 5, which is severe. Sometimes the scale is expanded to 10 which is very severe breathlessness.

Following this initial pre-rehab assessment, the five of us were ushered into a well-decorated conference room where tables had been set up in a large circle. A blackboard and screen in the front of the classroom including a video monitor was provided. This was our classroom.

Following introductions we were each given a three-ring notebook well organized with the ten specific lesson plans to be taught over a period of twelve sessions. We would meet twice weekly, Tuesdays and Thursdays, three and a half hours each day, from 1:00 P.M. to 4:30 P.M The first hour of class would be a regimen of measured exercise. The remaining time of one and a half hour was used for in-class training. On Thursdays this hour was used for a patient support group that was conducted and facilitated by a clinical social worker.

The textbook used was *Shortness of Breath; A Guide to Better Living and Breathing*, Fifth Edition, by Ries, Moser, Bullock, Limberg, Myers, Sassi-Dambron and Sheldon, 1996. Mosby-Year Book, Inc. A great COPD handbook!

The planned subjects for our study were: Orientation, Breathing Techniques, Exercise, Medications, Respiratory Concepts, Nutrition, When to Call your Doctor, Stress/Relaxation, and Travel.

## *Orientation*

Goals of the program were to: improve quality of life, reduce shortness of breath, improve exercise tolerance, and improve breathing techniques.

It is not my purpose in this writing to cover all the material I was fortunate to receive in rehabilitation training. What I wish to do is use my perceptions as a patient that I found most useful that profoundly changed my life.

It seems in any orientation session, one's impressions of what is about to happen to or with them and the other people in the class dominate their immediate interest. Two observations I made that first day in our orientation class have stayed in my mind ever since.

First of all, I quickly recognized that I was *not alone* in my dilemma of coping with lung disease. As I looked around the room, I was introduced to four other respiratory patients, that although different in our individual lives we were the same in this room this day, as our lives came together. I guess many people with disability recognize the humbling experience of empathy and mutuality when they realize they are not different from many others.

I learned something special from each of them, not just their particular coping skills that I could try, but also the way they each perceived their disability.

Jean is twenty years my senior and had never smoked. She is a very dignified and classy woman who had spent her life raising a family on a cattle and wheat ranch in rural Oregon. Very cultured and intelligent, even though she had never smoked, she somehow contracted COPD and was still managing to travel and spend quality time with her family. She was coping in a most productive way with her disease.

Dottie, also my senior by ten years, had worked hard all her life in many occupations, including years as a rural mail carrier from which she retired. Dottie had smoked all her life as I had and was now paying the price. Her daughter and granddaughter were her family. I watched her daughter smoke and continue to smoke cigarettes as she watched her mother deteriorate and struggle to breathe.

Bob was also many years my senior, coming from a huge family, a professional, educated farmer in rural Oregon. He was indeed a delightful man who had great stories about his days as a college baseball player. While managing his farm and orchards, Bob apparently had inhaled chemicals. One day he realized his lungs were so badly damaged he was disabled. In his final years he, like all of us, was without enough air to live his life.

Finally there was Fritz who was also my senior with whom I became good friends. Fritz smoked for many years as I did. He had been employed as a machinist requiring him to grind brake linings from which he inhaled asbestos causing him to suffer from *asbestosis*. You see, we were different, but in many ways also very much the same.

The second thing that I came away with that day of orientation that I have benefited from happens to be the Latin motto for one of our southern States. The motto reads, "Dum spiro, spero" and it means, *"While I breathe, I hope."* I found *new hope that I would get better*. I learned that I had some "control" over how I would cope with the progression of my lung disease.

A feeling of hopelessness and having no control over one's life is the main cause of depression. Depression is one's enemy when trying to cope with life because it actually distorts reality. It has been described to me as looking through distorted eyeglasses so that everything you see is altered from the reality that others may perceive it. This altered perception is most often negative and without hope. Hopelessness takes one on a downward spiral of negativism. If I got nothing else from that first day of orientation and introduction I got the message that I could improve the quality of my life. I had found hope.

I was not alone; there were new friends to learn from and I had hope that my life could get better if I was willing to make it happen with this new opportunity. My lungs were as bad, if not worse, than any other patient in the program that day. I had come to the right place for help. I was not alone. I would get better.

## Breathing Techniques

*"Smell the roses, blow out the candle"* has rung through my head hundreds of times the last few years during periods of severe

shortness of breath (dyspnea). This new breathing technique has literally kept me out of hospital emergency rooms. I had to relearn how to efficiently breathe with emphysema. Correct breathing is a natural phenomenon that begins when someone assaults your bottom or your feet just moments after you are born. After being born and slapped, poked, or prodded, you actively contracted your diaphragm, lifted your ribs and drew air into your previously collapsed, fluid-filled lungs for the first time. You announced your arrival into the world with a loud exhalation. By the time you were a teen you held your shoulders back and your stomach in and subsequently your breathing technique changed.

Using your diaphragm instead of your neck and shoulder muscles to breathe is more efficient and uses less oxygen. Therefore, there is more oxygen for your brain, heart, and other organs. Breathing is automatic but not any longer. With lung disease, one is conscious of his or her breathing most of the time. Correct breathing techniques are more efficient at getting oxygen distributed throughout the lungs and expelling carbon dioxide. I had to learn "pursed lip and diaphragmatic breathing." Every breath counts when one is out of air.

I say, *"The quality of our lives depends on the quality of our next breath."*

Think about it . . . it is true. I have been so out of air that I did not have enough breath to inhale bronchodilator medications to breathe better. My recovery depended on *"pursed lip breathing."* It is simple . . . just visualize: *"smell the rose, blow out the candle."* Breathe deep through your nose as if you smelled a rose, filling up your thoracic cavity full of air with your belly distended. Now purse your lips as if you are kissing or blowing a candle out and slowly blow all the air from your chest, sucking your belly in to force out any trapped air. Pursed lips create "back pressure" on your airways that actually hold them more open than usual, allowing a better flow of air.

Count to yourself while exhaling to establish a comfortable exhalation time.

Inhalation is just half of the count; exhalation is the second half. These counts become your paced breathing ratio. Many of us are comfortable inhaling for 2 counts and exhaling 4 counts, 2:4; some will prefer in for 2 and out 3 (2:3); others, inhaling for 3 and exhaling for 6 (3:6) You will know what you need.

When we get short of breath and feel as if we might suffocate, anxiety causes us to breathe fast and shallow when what we *need* to do is breathe slow and deep, maximizing our oxygen **in** and carbon dioxide **out**. This can only be accomplished by pursed lip diaphragmatic breathing . . . hence, *smell the rose, blow out the candle.*

You too can do this recovery breathing which can sometimes keep you from going to the hospital emergency room. Just as important, it can be used to keep one from not having enough air to walk a short distance or even enough breathe to inhale badly needed medication. Practicing this breathing method until it becomes second nature to us then requires less concentration and becomes an automatic rescue technique.

I have been told that some lung disease patients also develop Reactive Airway Disease (RAD), also referred to as "Hypersensitive Airways." This disease seems to be characterized by the patient developing a hypersensitivity to certain smells, toxins or airborne irritants that cause their airways to constrict, thereby obstructing the airflow. Pursed lip diaphragmatic breathing is useful whenever airflow is restricted for whatever reason. It takes me approximately two minutes to recover after I have run out of air. I refer to running out of air to my Janet as "crashing"; she then knows what is happening.

The diaphragm is the major muscle for inhalation. It actually is a large dome-shaped pair of muscles which rests just below the lungs, dividing the thoracic and abdominal cavities. The diaphragm is normally responsible for up to 80% of our breathing effort. Because of hyperinflation of the lungs, people with emphysema and bronchitis develop flattened diaphragms, which do not work efficiently to get air into and out of the lungs. The diaphragm can actually be somewhat reconditioned with exercise.

During inhalation, the diaphragm contracts, moving

downward, causing negative pressure inside the lungs. This negative pressure draws air into the lungs and equalizes the pressure. The downward diaphragmatic movement compresses the abdominal contents, causing the stomach to protrude slightly.

This is why diaphragmatic breathing is often called "belly breathing." I find it difficult to explain to someone who has not experienced this, but my lungs have hyperinflated so far down into my abdomen that just bending over or kneeling sometimes keeps me from breathing. When this occurs I actually feel my diaphragm stop moving or functioning. Often when severe, it feels like my diaphragm muscle actually cramps and has spasms like other muscles.

This is very painful and alarming when trying to breathe.

When this happens to me, I feel as though I will suffocate. I cannot get air moving in or out, I cannot inhale medication, and then panic begins to overtake my mind. It has taken years for me to learn to cope with this respiratory "crashing." By concentrating on *smelling the rose and blowing out the candle* it has become "okay" to be short of breath because I know that I can handle it. I now think of it as *"how to breathe when you can't."*

I know very well this is part of coping with emphysema. I know that I will get enough air with this new breathing technique I have learned. I do it every day of my life. My life depends on it.

Finding ways to more easily perform some of the required activities of daily living (ADL) becomes more and more essential. ADLs include eating, bathing, dressing, walking, lifting, etc. Here are some helpful ideas I learned to conserve my breath.

Plan your day to maximize your good breathing hours. Organize your time so you are not rushed and stressed to hurry in what you can do. Modify your activities, by sitting when possible, or using a cart with wheels to move heavy items. Eliminate tasks which are unnecessary and save steps in any way you can. Take short rest periods before you completely run out of air. Use a cordless phone to carry with you. Store items that you use often in a convenient place. Arrange your clothes and sit to dress and undress. Choose clothing that does not restrict your waist, wear slip on shoes with a comfortable fit. Use a waterproof seat with rubber tips in the shower or tub. Sit and use a handheld shower hose; use liquid soap. Sit while shaving. Plan small meals that minimize gas and restrict abdominal movement. There are many breath-saving methods I have learned from other COPD patients.

Having written the above, never stop doing what you can. I believe it is the wrong advice to tell a lung disease patient to "take it easy" and do not do activities if they are difficult. I have learned that *"if I do not try to do what I **can** then I do not know what I **can do!**"* Even if I "crash" while trying and need to recover from shortness of breath, I at least tried. If stairs are too high and too many, do what you can and rest. For example, you can water your lawn and have someone else mows it. Not trying to do what you can will be a definite deteriorating factor in your quality of life. I promise you that this is true.

## *Exercise*

On that cool, gray late November day in 1996 when I reported to pulmonary rehabilitation what I dreaded most was "exercise." I knew that I did not like exercise and it was one reason that I had never been particularly athletic. It was painful; no pain, no gain. I did not need pain. I had always been able to stay thin without exercise and now that I could not breathe and was fifty pounds heavier, how and why would I want to exercise? The six-minute assessment walk was almost impossible for me to get through as it was.

Wanda, the kind and supportive physical therapist who was there to help me, appeared to have more confidence in what I could do than I did. I started on one of the three treadmills with two of the other patients and began to walk one step at a time, slower then slower until the machine was turned down to .8 mph and continued to move my legs. After three minutes I had to stop and rest for a moment, then on for another three minutes. I was able to rest for two minutes and was then led to an Upper Body

Exerciser (UBE). I was seated, had the seat adjusted and began to turn the handles in a circle. After two minutes my arms began to ache but I continued for three minutes, rested and tried another minute then stopped. Each time an oximeter was used on my finger to measure my oxygen level and I was asked what my perceived breathlessness was on a scale from 1, being very slight to 5, being severe. I was never below 5 those first few sessions and was learning to pursed-lip breathe the entire time.

You may have noticed that some pulmonary patients try to compensate for their compromised breathing by using their shoulder and neck muscles. They can often be seen walking upright with their shoulders held up, shortening the appearance of their neck. What I eventually learned is that the muscles in my neck and shoulders were weak and I needed them for breathing.

When I was using my arms by raising them to shoulder level or above I could not use these same muscles to breathe with. They had become too weak and not available for both work and breathing. Exercise continued most of that session. I learned that we would eventually be expected to complete one hour of cumulative exercise on various pieces of equipment. Wanda said it would get easier. I trusted her.

I realized some important things that first week after I was introduced to exercise. Exercise must be seen as any other prescribed "medicine" taken daily to reduce adverse symptoms of my disease. I realized that I would need to lose some weight to improve my mobility. I was not going to improve my breathing very much and I knew from my days of dune buggy racing that if one cannot increase the horsepower of one's engine, then the weight of the dune buggy had to be reduced to be able to go faster. Seems simple; to have more power I would need less weight.

I further learned that the corticosteroids (prednisone) that I had been taking for six years had taken its toll on my body. I had added weight to my abdomen, my muscles had weakened, and my metabolism had changed, making me hungry and fat. I was fat and weak and needed to be lighter and stronger. This seemed simple, but was very difficult to make the transformation happen. I began the very long process of reducing my doses of prednisone. My goal would be to reactivate my natural production of this needed anti-inflammatory. It would take over a year to do this.

I had quit smoking by giving myself one year of change to see the results. I would give exercise a try to see the change. I went home that first week with a homework assignment of seven minutes of walking, five to ten minutes of rest then stretch-band stretching with my arms. I would give this effort a year by exercising daily, and with my doctor's approval, gradually reduce and eventually get off prednisone. The long process of withdrawal occurred a few milligrams at a time. Because of my difficulty in trying to breathe cold, dusty, hot, dry air, and too steep inclines, I decided to get a treadmill for my home exercise.

I could no longer make excuses to myself about the outside conditions. It was a very good, long-term decision. I put it in our guest room in view of the TV, where the scenery is changed with a click of the remote control.

I have endeavored to use that treadmill every day during the last five years; it will always remain part of my morning routine. I began increasing my daily exercise at pulmonary rehab and finally could do it for my one hour. I then began working on my weight and successfully lost one pound per week for the next year.

Exercise is the product we all need. I had heard it all my life and never realized how easily we are seduced into thinking we do not need exercise.

The less I do, the less I am able to do. Once I start slacking I feel less like exercising. By not using self-discipline and allowing myself to reduce my time from one hour to forty-five minutes, then I know it will be soon reduced to thirty minutes and so on, to become only fifteen minutes of exercise. Since the first and last five minutes are the most difficult, it makes it hard to get started. Once I get going my muscles seem to warm and tune up and it becomes easier. Each day I decide not to exercise, my body has a natural tendency towards unconditioning and relapsing to a state of nonconditioning.

To lose weight that first year I had to treadmill one hour per day at 2.0 mph.

Observe a patient in bed at rest for one week and see how weak their legs become. It is amazing what a few days of inactivity will do to the body.

After I lost fifty-plus pounds, I then reduced my exercise time to forty-five minutes daily. I then finally settled for thirty minutes each day at 2.0 mph or one mile per day for the last few years. I could easily reduce this to twenty minutes daily but I refuse to. At thirty minutes each day, I must watch my caloric intake to maintain my 152-pound, thirty-two-inch waist on my five-foot-ten-inch medium body frame. I can immediately recognize any weight gain and the difference it makes on my mobility with my lung capacity. In my opinion, it is almost impossible to lose weight in a healthy way without exercising.

Exercise has become part of my life style included in my daily routine. Sitting in a chair doing upper body-chair exercises is better than no exercise. Walking seems to be the best, most effective, exercise effort for the amount of time spent. It is available and free for everyone. Thirty minutes of walking exercise each day, four days a week, will maintain my condition. Five to seven days a week will build and improve my physical condition. The very best investment for my health has been my electric treadmill.

For most of us, weight is determined by how many calories our body is consuming compared to how many calories our body needs to burn for our level of activity. There are, of course, exceptions, but fewer than people think. Try carrying around a five or ten-pound bag of sugar or even a twenty-five-pound bag of dog food the next time you are shopping at a grocery store.

Carrying a bag of extra weight will quickly show you how much more your body must work to carry excess weight.

One of the unhealthiest conditions for a person with lung disease is to be obese. An extra twenty to one hundred pounds of weight for weak lungs to support takes a very negative toll on COPD patients. I carried an extra fifty pounds and was able to experience the difference in my capacity for exercise. I never want to go through the effort it took to lose that weight again. I have learned that the quality of my physical ability to do every activity in my daily life, as well as control my weight, is directly related to my willingness to do my daily treadmill exercise. The less I exercise, the less walking I can enjoy when the opportunity arises. It is all a matter of choice.

Daily exercise has become a scheduled priority. I need to constantly protect this priority or it doesn't happen for me. Other activities very easily can interfere with the time I have set aside for this needed exercise. "Those who think they have no time for daily exercise will sooner or later have to find time for illness."

## A Product: By Catherine McNeil

*If* you could purchase a product which could cut your risk of dying from heart disease by 50 percent; and . . .

*If* this product were also a major factor in the prevention and cure of diabetes, arthritis, osteoporosis, insomnia, obesity and hypertension; and . . .

*If* this product reduced resting heart rate, lowered blood pressure, increased metabolic efficiency, lowered blood cholesterol and, in terms of the most fundamental physiological measure, seemed able to retard and, in some cases reverse the aging process; and . . .

*If* this product made you leaner, lighter, firmer, shapelier, stronger and more flexible, agile, mobile, alert, energetic, confident, optimistic, and, last but not least, more attractive; and . . .

*If* this same product reduced stress, alleviated depression, relaxed anxiety, dissipated anger, raised the spirits, enhanced self-esteem, improved concentration and relaxed body, mind; and . . .

*If* this product were associated with eating better and eating less, consuming less alcohol, smoking less tobacco and, in general, having more control over one's life; and . . .

*If*, as a result of using this product, men and women in every profession had more stamina and staying power, were ill less frequently and less seriously and possessed more energy, creativity and optimism than their sedentary colleagues; and . . .

*If* it were becoming better known every year that the value of this product, while important at every age, became more important as men and women advanced from their thirties into their forties, fifties, sixties and beyond; and . . .

*If*, moreover, these claims for this product came not from advertising agencies, but rather from university laboratories, scientific journals and independent research analysis . . .

Then, would you be interested in using this product regularly?

## The Product is *Exercise!*

### *Medications*

*First of all: Before making any changes in your medications, diet, exercise or alternative methods of treatments . . . consult your doctor.*

The word medicine comes from Latin *medicina* and *medicus* for physician.

A dictionary may define medicate as "to treat with medicine" and medicine as "any substance or substances used in treating disease or illness."

The art or science of *diagnosing, treating or preventing disease* based on this definition, "medication" could include drugs, nebulizers, diet or special foods, sanitation of inhalation equipment preventing infection, exercise, and even mental health techniques to improve the way we think about illness.

For the purpose of sharing my perspective of COPD associated medications, I will start with the chemical medications I was taking during my pre-pulmonary rehabilitation days and into the first year of rehabilitation.

Since 1993 and of course during the preceding three years,

I had seen seven different physicians, three of them specialists, two practicing in pulmonary medicine.

During the last ten years, I have had prescribed to me the following medications to treat the symptoms of COPD and other related problems.

It is a very common fact that many patients are "over-medicated" especially the elderly. Look at this list of medications that I have "tried:"

Acetaminophen, Advil, Aerobid, metered dose inhaler meds (MDI), Alupent MDI, Atrovent MDI, Azmacort MDI, Albuterol Sulfate MDI, Amoxil, Augmentin, Biaxin, Buspar, Cardura, Ceftin, Centrum Silver, Cephalexin, Cyclobenzaprin, Combivent MDI, Deltasone, Doxcycl, Flovent MDI, HCTZ, Hytrin, Nebulizer both PulmoAide and Ultrasonic with a transducer, Orasone, prednisone (with daily doses for five years), Prometh SYP, Proscar, Provental Retab, Robitussin Expectorant, Serevent, SMZ TMP, Sulfamethox, Theodur (Theophylline for 5 years without a blood level monitoring) Voltex, Xanax, Xopenex, Zithromax, and Zoloft.

It is a very wise treatment practice, once each year, for every patient to put all their medications, vitamins, inhalers, and any other treatments they are using in a bag and bring them to their doctor's appointment and ask their doctor to reconfirm that it is okay to continue consuming the cumulative combination of drugs. This practice could save one's life or identify toxic side effects they may be suffering from.

I carefully consider needed changes in my medical regimen . . . "It is just as important to change medicine if needed as it may be **not** to change what is working well." Actually I am careful about taking any medication; every action has a reaction of some kind; every substance you put in your body has some kind of reaction or effect, and it may be negative.

This consideration is especially important in an older person with a changed metabolism and perhaps compromised immune system. It is desirable for us now to ask our physicians to start at the lowest dose possible when starting a new medication to see how it will react with our body then gradually increase it if necessary. These practices are much safer than taking a normal or higher dose as prescribed then needing to decrease it when you notice problems or when your doctor may or may not ask you if the medications are working. I have had three different physicians prescribe anti-depressants and leave me on the same dose for nine months to a year without ever talking to me about possibly adjusting the dose or monitoring the effect. In each case, I carefully and gradually discontinued the medication and found out it was not having the desired effect on me for which it was prescribed. As a matter of fact, I was having negative effects such as blunting (dulling) of emotions and reduced libido (interest in sex) from the medication, Zoloft, with no positive effects. It seems that I had spent nine months of unnecessary medication on this one case and there are other examples I could give. It is imperative to monitor the effects of any prescribed medication to know if you are taking *the minimum amount needed to achieve the maximum benefit.* Everyone is an individual and may react and use medications differently. You are always "Yo-Yo" (**Y**ou're **O**n **Y**our **O**wn) to manage your own medications.

A fellow COPD patient, Bill Horden, once wrote in his *COPD Survival Guide:*

On the Internet: "I've got to warn you against the temptation that when you are getting good results from your new medication, your improved diet and your exercise, to alter the routine or skip a day. Remember, it was this regimen and this routine that produced the improvement; stay with it unless your doctor says otherwise. Don't let success ruin your good work." He gives good advice on this issue.

By the time I had been under treatment for COPD for six years I had been introduced to many different antibiotics, bronchodilators, and corticosteroids. Also I had tried many different inhalers, spacers, and nebulizers. Learning about these new medications was getting confusing and difficult.

During my training as a Navy Hospital Corpsman in the late 50's I became interested in my pharmacology classes. I learned that medications have very specific uses and contraindications for nonuse.

During my twenty-five years in law enforcement I had seen the devastating use of illegal and prescription drugs.

We kept a *Physicians Desk Reference* (PDR) in our sheriff's office and were constantly trying to identify pills and capsules of medications we found abused on the street. I was interested in the names and composition of drugs and read the enclosed insert on my prescribed medications for possible side effects. So when I was getting confused about all the medications I was taking, many without much information, it made me a bit uncomfortable.

One of the physicians that I saw along the way of seeking relief from my emphysema symptoms told me about National Jewish Medical and Research Center located in Denver, Colorado.

This medical center was and is still a national leader in lung, allergic and immune diseases. *U.S. News and World Report* reported the National Jewish Medical and Research Center as the number one respiratory hospital in America for the last five years. My doctor spoke of their COPD treatment class to teach patients how to manage their lung condition. He further explained this two-week class was offered only in Denver and that my medical insurance probably would not pay for it. He was correct, it would not be paid for, and I would not go.

This helpful doctor offered to loan me his 45-minute tape cassette recording of the basics in managing your lung condition from one of the Jewish Medical Center classes. I borrowed it, copied it, learned from it and shared these tips with hundreds of other lung patients. Many years passed and much good was done from this tape.

Last year I was attending a health foundation philanthropy conference in Santa Fe and met the executive officer and program director of National Jewish Medical and Research Center. I got tears in my eyes as I explained to him how valuable his outreach program had been to me and hundreds of other struggling COPD patients in America. It is truly amazing how we are all connected.

This Jewish Medical Center cassette tape begins with the recording physician explaining the anatomy and physiology of diseased lungs. The physician recording the tape explains the constricted obstructed airways including the inflammation that causes phlegm and wheezing which was then referred to as "Chronic Airway Disease." The physician recording the tape outlines the three goals of the program at the National Jewish Hospital as:

1. *For the patient to learn everything possible about their lung disease, they must manage it themselves and use their physician as a consultant.*

2. *To achieve the most wide open airways possible (FEV1) using the minimum amount of medication.*

3. *Increase the patient's ability to perform physical activity, overcoming any fear of exertion or reluctance to exercise.*

All three of these goals are worthy of consideration, especially in the prevention and treatment of lung disease.

He further explained the regimen of COPD medications in a way that I first began to understand as the ABC's of lung disease treatment. He continues to emphasize *taking the minimum dose to achieve the maximum benefit.*

The ABC's of respiratory treatment medications he described are:

Aminophylline (theophylline family) prescribed first to open airways.

Beta-2 agonists (bronchodilators) prescribed second if needed to open airways.

Corticosteroids (anti-inflammatory) prescribed to reduce inflammation.

Some of the objectives of my pulmonary rehabilitation medication class were to understand the side effects of breathing medications, actively participate in managing my medications, and learn to use my pharmacist as a member of my treatment consultant team.

I had taken aminophylline (Theodur) for approximately five years and in that time received only one blood level test. This test is really important to determine the level of medication in a patient's blood. I had gradually been elevated in dose until I was on 1200 to 1500 mg daily. This medication may help many chronic lung disease patients, but I knew of the side effects and one was causing me to feel "jittery," I was already jittery from the Albuterol I was taking. I asked my doctor if I could try to discontinue this medication. He agreed so I began to taper the dose and finally stopped taking it. For me, I noticed *no significant difference* in the way I was able to breath or perform the physical activities of rehab exercise. I felt liberated from one medication and began to evaluate others.

For the purposes of simplification, and knowing most of the severely disabled COPD people I know use antibiotics for lung infections, I changed the "A" in the ABC equation to stand for antibiotics.

To further simplify discussing medications with new COPD people who are really intimidated by new, long, hard to pronounce, medical terms, I changed Beta 2 Agonist to just plain "Bronchodilators." Corticosteroids completes the ABCs of COPD medications.

Now knowing how I got to this acronym, and that it may not be technically correct, one can see that it is easier to learn. A is for Antibiotics, B is for Bronchodilators, and C is for Corticosteroids. Since learning is best "caught," not "taught" in small bites or pieces of information, I have had good results in using this explanation for new COPD patients.

As a personal practice I have learned to ask myself these questions regarding any medication I decide to take into my body:

What is the name, including generic and brand names, of the medication?

Why am I taking this medicine; is it at the minimum amount necessary?

How am I supposed to take this medication to receive maximum benefit?

## Antibiotics

There continues to be new antibiotics on the market. It is prudent to understand that the overuse of antibiotics can result in your body not benefiting as much from them when a more severe bacterial infection occurs.

Some cautious physicians I observe seem reluctant to prescribe antibiotics for beginning lung infections. We know that one's lungs are the perfect place for bacteria to grow and thrive. The lung environment is dark, warm, and moist. Diseased lung tissue lacks an adequate blood and air supply, allowing an even more ideal place for bacteria to survive and infection to linger. Although viruses can lead to the most common lung infections, antibiotics are not effective against virus. Antibiotics used against typical post-viral bacteria are thought to be beneficial. Antibiotics either kill the intruding bacteria, or stop the replication of the bacteria so that the human body's natural defenses can kill the bacteria.

Most COPD patients that are on corticosteroids may have a compromised immune system that does not fight bacteria very well and must not be treated the same as a person with a normal immune system. When I begin to recognize I may be getting a lung infection, I pay close attention to the symptoms. If it is a common cold, the initial phlegm from my lungs is not colored, although copious and congested, it remains fairly clear. A lung infection will be easily recognized by the color of phlegm changing from clear to yellow, to brown, to nasty tasting blebs from deep in your chest. When the phlegm color changes, I get concerned and immediately call my doctor. All too often it occurs on a Friday and waiting to get started on an antibiotic is not a good thing. For me, waiting two or three days can mean two or three month's recovery time.

Many medical centers and private doctor's offices, to reduce costs, now use "medical technicians," not registered nurses. They are often the person who decides who gets in to see the doctor. When a patient with severe emphysema calls their doctor and they are told to "take some Aspirin or Aleve and let us know how you feel in a week," I say, "change docs." This happens too often. If my efforts to get started on an antibiotic fail, especially on a holiday or long weekend, I may go to a Care-Clinic or Emergency Room. I just do not wait "a few days to see if I am better." Antibiotics are promptly needed to stop the lung infection from advancing possibly into pneumonia.

Each of us should know if we have any allergies and remember to tell our doctor when deciding to use antibiotics. I have had physicians that trusted me to know when I needed an antibiotic, and let me keep a stand-by prescription to use in emergency situations. It was wonderful and very efficient for me.

I have learned that it is important to take all the prescribed medication even after I begin to feel better or the phlegm clears up. The infections will linger and if all the antibiotic medication is not utilized, it may re-occur. I always follow the directions and notes on the prescription bottle.

"It is a good thing to do." Some of the common antibiotics used for lung infections are:

| Generic | Brand |
|---|---|
| amoxicillin | Amoxil |
| ampicillin | Omniven |
| amoxicillin-potassium | Augmentin |
| azithromycin | Zithromax |
| ciprofloxacin | Cipro |

There are many more very effective antibiotics and more coming on to the pharmaceutical market every year.

## Bronchodilators

*(Simply means to open airways.)*

For simplification, I will include the anticholinergic agent (atropine), generic ipratropium bromide, brand name "Atrovent" in this category. Technically, this medication works a little differently than true bronchodilators as it blocks specific receptors found in the lung that promote constriction of the airways. Today this medication is most often combined with the beta 2 agonist to form the "rescue" and airway dilator prescription medication most of us take. The medication inhaler, (Metered Dose Inhaler or MDI), named Combivent is a good example. If one is taking both albuterol sulphate and Atrovent in two different inhalers (MDI's), it is much more convenient and cost effective to use the combination of both meds in one as in a Combivent inhaler.

The bronchodilator medication inhaler that almost all COPD patients use or have used is a critical medication to know about. It is the medication that is carried in our shirt or trouser pocket, jacket, purse, glove box, or a spare in the garage or shop. This medication is the one your significant other, spouse, kids, neighbor or anyone else, needs to know to get for you when you cannot. It is my "rescue" medication. It is so important that I use a happy-face sticker placed on the end of the canister so my wife can get the correct one for me when I cannot talk. It is the inhaler that I worry about, when I do not have enough breath to inhale it deep into my lungs. It is the one I take as prescribed whether I need it when it is time or not, and "before" I get in trouble. I take it before I exercise or before I engage in any activity. It is the medication I do not overdose on because I know if I use too much it may not work as effectively when I really need it. It relaxes and opens my airways and keeps me from suffocating. *It is always taken first and before steroids.*

Here are the names of some I have used:

| Generic | Brand |
|---------|-------|
| albuterol sulphate | Albuterol, Provental, Ventolin |
| bitolterol | Tornalate |
| metaproterenol | Alupent, Metaprel |
| pirbuterol | Maxair |
| terbutaline | Breathair, Brethine, Bricanyl |

## Metered Dose Inhalers (MDI)

I incorrectly used and watched other people incorrectly use inhalers for many years.

*The maximum benefit of any medication can only be achieved if the medications are administered properly.*

A metered dose inhaler is in fact a canister of medication usually measured in gram weight of medication under the pressure of a propellant. Each time one depresses the canister into the holder, it depresses the pressure value allowing a "dose" to be released from the mouthpiece. This simply requires careful coordination, which takes practice to synchronize the release of medication at exactly the correct time, allowing it to be inhaled slowly and deeply through the airways and deep into the patient's lungs.

Each canister usually holds from 120 to 200 actuations or dose inhalations of medication. This amount is clearly printed on the canister. If the medication is prescribed for "two puffs, four times daily" as Combivent and Albuterol are prescribed, the canister should last (200 divided by 8 = 25 days) twenty-five days. This is important because most medical insurance companies will only fill one every month or 30 days. A patient will struggle with having enough medication to last a month if they do not get the physician to write, "use two puffs every four hours as needed" on the prescription. A patient using Flovent, a very important corticosteroid that should never be abruptly stopped, will have 120 doses in a MDI canister. Corticosteroids are usually prescribed 2 puffs twice daily, (120 divided by 4 =

30) thirty days for each canister. Steroid medication should *not* be carried around in one's pocket with the rescue inhaler; instead it should be kept by their bed or kitchen table where it is used only twice daily; in the morning when they get up and at night before bedtime.

One can then mark thirty days from when they open a new box of medication and know about when they will be "out" of medication. Sometimes I will write, using black ink "Sharpie" pen, the start date on the side of the canister holder. A very acceptable method of measuring the amount of medication left in an MDI canister is to "float" it in a cup of water. Since the medication is measured by weight, if it is full it will sink, if it is half-full it will float. With approximately one-half of the canister submerged in the water, if it is empty, it will float on its side on top of the water. When the medication canister is empty (floating on its side) discard it.

Recently, the manufactures of some metered dose inhalers are advising users *not to submerge the canisters in water.* I have submerged hundreds of canisters, hundreds of times, I have never had a problem doing this that I know of. It is always better to error on the side of discarding your canister too soon, than to use it when it is empty. I am open to new information and have been told that each canister medication may "float differently" and the float method of determining the amount of medication in a canister is not reliable.

Whichever method you choose, carefully measure the remaining contents of your medication inhaler canisters often especially when they are nearly empty.

In an attempt to protect the environment, by not using propellants in the medication canister, many manufactures are now dispensing some of these medications in a "diskus." A diskus is medication in an enclosed plastic disc, containing 60 tiny packets of powder (2 puffs daily for 30 days). One packet is ruptured at a time, allowing the patient to inhale the medicated powder into their lungs without the use of a propellant. When inhaling medication, you must inhale slowly and deeply into the small airways of your lungs. If inhaled to quickly the medication will be drawn into the large airways and never get into the small areas where it is needed most. Small particles deliver smaller droplets of medication to the lungs. A "spacer" is critical to assist in doing this.

## Spacers

I have used many different kinds of spacers. Some were large, expensive, hard to clean, and cumbersome to conveniently carry. Consequently, I did not use one as most of the other COPD patients I notice do not either. On the tape cassette I listened to from the National Jewish Medical Center I learned about using a piece of plastic respiratory tubing about 5/8" in diameter and 4" long stuck on the mouthpiece of an inhaler. A six-inch piece comes with most nebulizer packets and every hospital respiratory department has hundreds of feet of this respiratory tubing. Since I have started using this type of spacer I would not consider using an inhaler without one. I have a mustache and cannot imagine holding my inhaler 2" to 3" from my mouth and spraying the medication over my chin, lips and teeth as suggested by some "instructions" I have seen.

The purpose of a spacer is to let the large particles drop out of the dispensed inhaler to the bottom of the spacer, allowing the smaller droplets to be deeply inhaled into your lungs. It does work and helps keep the medication off your tongue, teeth, moustache and face. Most important of all, a spacer will keep inhaled medication from accidentally getting in your eyes. Always rinse your mouth after taking any inhaled medication, especially corticosteroids.

There are those who will argue that other types of spacers are better, more effective, and should be used. A spacer will not work no matter how good it is if you do not have it with you when taking your inhaled medication. I want every inhaler user to use a spacer. If you will at least try a piece of tubing it will be better than not using a spacer. Actually I have heard COPD patients tell me they have used an empty toilet paper cardboard tube for a spacer. I tried the toilet paper tube, it works fine. That is why the piece of plastic tubing is so valuable. I take a 6-inch piece, cut it in half making two 3-inch pieces, using a different spacer for each inhaler. They will fit in pockets, purses, jackets and even the box the medication comes in. If someone wanted to, they could use this plastic tube spacer as a "disposable" item, discarding it when it needed cleaning. They cost less than a dollar to make.

My wife Janet and I used all the plastic tubing we could get from our local medical center respiratory department and made hundreds of packets of two spacers and gave them to every new pulmonary rehabilitation patient that came to the program. We made more and gave them to every doctor in town to recommend that their patient use them. We named them the "JP" spacer (my wife's initials). We then got a respiratory tubing company in California to donate 200 feet of tubing to us for this use. Janet and I then made up 400 more spacers, packaged them in special-sized, zip lock bags, just the perfect size container for two spacers and two inhalers. By heating the plastic tubing in warm water, these spacers will fit on both round and oval-size mouthpieces. We gave these spacers away free to any patient we could get to try a spacer, over 600 total, never charged one cent for them. I wish the inhaler manufactures would include such a device in each new inhaler box.

## *Ther Correct Way To Use An Inhaler*

Pick up and look at the medicated inhaler, hold it up and read the label to make sure it is the correct medication. I was taught to do this in the Navy Hospital Corps. It is a good habit to get into with all medications you are taking. Store each medication with the label out, and always hold it up and read the label before dispensing.

This is the only opportunity you will have to keep yourself from taking the wrong medication. Shake the inhaler to mix up the medication and if you have not used it for a few days or if it is a new canister, press the canister down for a "test" blast puff, making sure your spacer is in place.

Get ready for the medication by making room for it in your lungs. Exhale all the air using diaphragmatic (belly) and pursed lip breathing (*blow out the candle*) until you have drawn your stomach in forcing all the air from your chest. As you get ready to slowly and steadily inhale deep into your lungs, place the end of the spacer between your teeth and depress the canister all the way down. As the medication is dispensed begin your inhalation. When your inhalation is complete, hold your breath for a few seconds allowing the medication to be fully dispensed. Slowly exhale and resume normal breathing. After waiting a few minutes (two to four) repeat the procedure for the "second puff."

Remember: *"The effectiveness of your inhaled medications will never be better than your willingness and ability to use the inhaler as directed above." Which one will quickly learn . . . and then from ones medication "The quality of your life depends on the quality of your next breath."*

Understanding that the most effective inhaled medication is going to be in small particles or droplets, it is plain to see that using a nebulizer is the very best method to change a liquid medication to a vapor for inhalation.

A nebulizer is simply a compressor that compresses air and forces it through a hose to a chambered device holding a liquid medication that can changed and inhaled as a gas or vapor.

There are many different brands of nebulizers, in both stationary and portable models. Ultrasonic nebulizers use a transducer medication cup heated electrically, which dispenses a vapor for inhalation. I have used both and prefer the air compressor which is virtually trouble free. This method requires the patient to sit and breathe slowly; it usually takes 15 minutes for one medication and 25 to 30 minutes for the two mixed medications in a sterile saline solution. I use Albuterol and Atrovent, which are frequently used together.

There seems to be very differing physician's opinions on the effectiveness of the inhaler versus the daily use of nebulizers. There is continuing controversy and ongoing research to study evidence indicating that an inhaler may be equally as effective as a nebulizer. If this were true the emergency rooms across the country would be using inhalers (MDI) for patients in respiratory distress instead of the nebulizer method of administering emergency breathing medications.

A breathing mask is also available if needed while using a nebulizer. It seems to me just sitting quietly and deeply breathing medications in the form of a very fine mist for ten to fifteen minutes is more effective that a quick inhalation of two puffs from an inhaler. I use a nebulizer at home and carry a rescue inhaler if needed in my car. It seems to be the best of both worlds.

One other consideration on nebulizer use is the fact that Medicare pays for nebulizer and nebulizer-dispensed respiratory medications. Medicare does not pay for inhalers. I use $1,000.00 worth of medications monthly. I am grateful for the Medicare assistance with my medication costs.

One other thing I learned is how very important cleaning all inhalers and nebulizer equipment is in preventing lung infections. At the end of each day I disassemble and wash my nebulizer medication holder parts in hot soapy dishwashing liquid and let it air dry for the next day. At the end of each week, I wash everything including all inhalers, holders, spacers, and medication nebulizer "bongs." I soak them in hot soapy water, use a toothbrush which just fits perfectly to brush clean the inside of spacers and canister holders. The accumulated medication residual one may see in the canister mouthpiece and spacer is good evidence that the spacer is doing its job.

Using a spacer will keep this medication off your face and trap the large particles inside the spacer, allowing the smaller ones to flow to your lungs. I scrub the residual medications off both the canister holder and spacer each week with a toothbrush after it has been soaking in soapy water; rinse, then sterilize in a white vinegar solution and reuse them usually for the period the canister lasts—30 days.

All my medication dispensers get soaked a second time in a mixture of nature's most effective sterilizer, white vinegar; about one part vinegar to two parts water for at least two hours, rinse in warm water and air dry.

By religiously cleaning and sterilizing my respiratory equipment this way I have reduced my lung infections by at least 50%. Storage of all clean, contaminate-free respiratory equipment can be accomplished by using a meat loaf size Tupperware type container.

I use the same method for my other daily medications, including a daily/weekly tablet box. This keeps me from forgetting if I have taken a daily dose of meds and to manage the reordering when necessary. I also use a small freezer zip lock bag for the inhalers and spacers that I carry in my car, etc. This system easily keeps them clean and dust-free.

Mouth hygiene becomes especially important to those of us frequently inhaling medications into our mouths and on our tongues. Frequent rinsing and hydrating with water is essential. Toothbrushes should be used daily to brush the medication off our tongues and prevent mouth yeast infections named "thrush" from occurring.

After being sick with a cold or the flu, toothbrushes should always be changed to keep from re-infecting yourself.

## Corticosteroids

Corticosteroids are synthetically produced in medications used primarily as anti-inflammatory agents for inflamed lungs or bronchitis (inflammation of the bronchi). The cassette tape previously indicated from National Jewish Medical Center suggested that steroids were too often prescribed "too little too late" and for "too long of a period of time." It suggested that a more appropriate use for acute exacerbations of lung infections is to prescribe a higher dose for a shorter time then taper and discontinue as soon as possible.

After the initial large dose of prednisone, the medication can sometimes be slowly and gradually tapered off during the next two weeks. Long-term use of 5 to 30 mg per day for months or even years should be seriously considered and justified. The practice of taking this medication every other day reduces the side effects.

Sometimes taking these medications every third day, if possible, lessens harmful side effects.

The use of an inhaled steroid is less harmful than when taken orally (systemic).

Because of the potential for adverse effects, long-term treatment is usually only used for patients with definite improvement in air flow or exercise performance.

*The most important goal is to use only the amount of monitored steroid necessary to achieve the maximum benefit.*

I found that it is critical for each of us to manage ourselves using our doctor as a consultant. Side effects of the inhaled steroids mostly involve the overall body and there are many.

*Abrupt withdrawal of any steroid can be life threatening because our body has temporarily lost its ability to make natural steroids. Discuss any medication changes with your physician or pharmacist!*

A group called G.A.S.P. (Group Action Into Steroid Prescribing) by A.L.E.R.T. (Allied Lawyers Response Team) in July 1998 provided this list on the super highway of information: an Internet Web site, "Side-Effects of Prescribed Corticosteroid Drugs" . . . Just for your information:

> *Damage to the nervous system (I am dealing with neopathy*
> *in my feet)*
> *Heart Failure*
> *Kidney Failure*
> *Diabetes*
> *Osteoporosis (brittle bones)*
> *Mood Swings (I have to deal with acrophobia and*
> *irritability)*
> *Depression (I have experienced unexplained periods of*
> *depression)*

*Cataracts (I have both eye lenses replaced from cataracts at age sixty-two)*

*Glaucoma*

*Eye Problems*

*Weight Gain (I gained and had to lose fifty-two pounds)*

*Food Cravings*

*Moon Face (I have had and lost this fat face look)*

*Buffalo Hump (on back)*

*Headaches (I treat headaches nightly)*

*Bruising (I continue to see dark bruise patches on my hands and arms)*

*Pain in back and legs*

*Acne*

*Stretch Marks*

*Memory Loss (I have noticed short-term loss)*

*Muscle Weakness (Steroids make you fat and weak, not lean and strong)*

*Fluid Retention (I eventually needed to use a diuretic)*

*Period Problems/Early Menopause*

*Facial Hair Growth (Women)*

*Poor/Slow Healing Process*

*Teeth and Gum Problems*

*High Blood Pressure*

*High Blood Cholesterol*

*Swollen Hands and Ankles*

*Thinning Skin (you can easily see the tissue-paper skin on us steroid users)*

*Bowel Problems*

*Excessive Sweating*

*Avascular Necrosis*

*Loss of Sex Drive (libido)*

*Insomnia*

*Stomach Ulcers*

*Angina/Heart Problems*

*Body Cramps (I deal with feet and lower leg cramps nightly)*

*Indigestion/Heart Burn*
*Change in Composition/Strength of toe/finger nails*
*Hair Breaking/Hair Loss*
*Psychosis (very rare and seldom occurs but most alarming)*
*Suppression and destruction of the body's immune system*

Beginning during the year1997, while in rehab and with my doctor's assistance, I also began the very long process of reducing my doses of prednisone. I hoped to reactivate my natural production of this needed anti-inflammatory. It would take fourteen months to transition to inhaled corticosteroids. The withdrawal of systemic prednisone taken orally by tablet was painful and difficult. I was able to be weaned down to 2 mg every other day, and then went on the inhaled (MDI) corticosteroid called Flovent (Fluticasone propinate). Flovent can be prescribed in three strengths 220 mcg, 110 mcg, and 44 mcg at 2 puffs twice daily; 120 inhalations per canister.

This process took fourteen months! It was essential for me to slowly decrease the doses a few milligrams at a time, at two-week intervals then finally substituting the inhaled corticosteroids for the steroid tablets. I am told one's adrenal glands can produce approximately 7 mg of natural anti-inflammatory steroids on their own. What happens to people who take and continue to use corticosteroids for a period of years is that they become "steroid-dependent," which means their own adrenal glands stop producing natural steroids and become dependant on the medication. I am steroid dependant and will always need some to fight the inflammation of my lungs.

On occasion I have misjudged the number of doses in my Flovent inhaler. At the end of the calculated period of use (4 puffs daily x 30 days = 120 doses), i.e., on the thirtieth day, keep checking the contents daily, if necessary to avoid using an empty canister. In just three days I began feeling weak, noticed joint pain, and began an actual exacerbation of my COPD from the lack of this medication. It is not wise to "run out" or stop this medication abruptly.

I know I am taking the "minimum amount of corticosteroids to give me the maximum amount of benefit." I keep testing this so I "know."

If you are taking this medication you need to find out if you are taking the minimum amount that you need. Corticosteroids (prednisone) are magic drugs. When your lungs are inflamed and you are having an exacerbation of lung problems, this medication is magic but the good comes with bad side effects.

## Some Commonly Prescribed Corticosteriods:

| Generic | Brand |
|---|---|
| (Inhalation) | |
| beclomethasone | Beclovent |
| | Vanceril |
| triamcinolone | Azmacort |
| flunisolide | AeroBid |
| fluticasone propionate | Flovent (220, 110, and 44 mcg) |
| (Oral) | |
| methylprednisolone | Medrol |
| prednisolone | Delta-Cortef |
| prednisone | Deltasone, Orasone |
| triamcinolone | Aristocort, Kenacort |

By losing weight (over fifty pounds) and countering the bad side effects of prednisone after the first year of exercise, I became a different person in a different body. I was now encouraged to continue my effort and avoid that level of disability as long as possible.

Determining maximum desired benefit from medication taken is usually related to level of physical activity. For some it will be the degree of shortness of breath, for others it will be determined by lung volume test numbers. Still others desire a complete battery of pulmonary function tests (PFT) and arterial blood gas (ABG) measurement.

For clarification and definition, the test "forced expiratory volume in one second," (FEV1) measures the patient taking the deepest breath possible, then blowing out as much of that breath as possible in one second. FVC is the abbreviation for "forced vital capacity." It is measured in the same way as the FEV1. The patient exhales as rapidly and completely as possible, but the one-second time limit is not used.

FRC is the abbreviation for "functional residual capacity." It refers to the amount of air remaining in the lungs at the end of a normal breath. This test is significant in measuring volume in emphysema patients.

Tidal volume is the quantity of air inhaled and exhaled in one breath of normal breathing.

I often observe COPD patients comparing their FEV1/FVC numbers to compare levels of disability. I have done it myself. Sometimes I have noticed what appears to be an oversimplification and even a justification of activity based on one's test "numbers." After many years of various testing methods, I find myself using a subjective quality of life level of activity that I know works for me. It is how I "feel" and *how well I am able to accomplish the activities of daily living (ADL) that really determine my level of disability.* Perceived breathlessness is subjective and is only an indicator of lung volume.

Some of us learn to tolerate breathlessness more than others. Some are unable to overcome the fear of exertion and remain reluctant to exercise at all. I do better than some and not as well as others. My numbers are quite low; I do well with what I have. I am grateful for the good days I have.

Having shared the above information, I need to say that it is from my experiences and based on my observations. I have indeed used the medications and equipment listed. There will be some who will disagree with what I have said. There will be those who will challenge my opinion on the management of my disease and they are also correct. It is what works for each person that needs to be found.

# Chapter 5

## Pulmonary Rehabilitation—
## The Mind and Spirit

*"What we think, or what we know, or what we believe is, in the end, of little consequence. The only consequence is what we do."*

*John Ruskin*

In 1999, two full years after I had completed pulmonary rehabilitation, I received a letter from my doctor. She was leaving her practice in my area; it was definitely my loss, I miss her. She was definitely one of the most caring and compassionate physicians I've been fortunate to have. She had introduced me to the treatment for severe emphysema, lung volume reduction surgery screening, and transplantation evaluation. She was the physician that prescribed and supported my efforts in completing pulmonary rehabilitation. I always felt as if I was an important patient to her. She would listen to what I had to say; and it seemed important to her.

She wrote a farewell letter to all her patients that read in part:

*Always remember: You are in control of your health. I have only been the vessel through which you have gained knowledge to accomplish that end.*

I will always remember this bit of wisdom from her that I learned early in managing my disability.

From *Dictionary.com*: *Spirit* is Middle English, from Old French *espirit*, from Latin *spritus*, *breath*, from sprre, *to breathe*. It was when I learned that the word "breath" comes from the word "spirit" that I first began to make the mind-body connection. Some say that Genesis, chapter 1 of the Bible actually begins with the "wind"; breath or Spirit of God sweeping over the face of the water to start the creation of the Universe. We know that human life begins with the cry of first breath. We know that the last breath frequently determines the pronouncement of death. We know medically when determining what serious injury to treat first, that physicians, EMT rescue, emergency room staff, and first aid personnel treat stopped breathing before bleeding. I further learned that in meditation and relaxation techniques one's breathing could control the actual rate of blood pressure and pulse.

Ancient Eastern culture has written much on the yin and yang and the center of Chi (energy). Many other ancient cultures included body-soul recognition in the treatment of illness and injury. Much is written on this mind-body connection. We can then say breath is the Alpha and Omega of life, the beginning and the end. Breathing and how we control it is a very clear factor of health and our mind has more control over our body than most of us think.

In the works of Socrates I read that the very early teaching physicians in Florence, Greece, over 2000 years ago taught "Sickness of the mind makes the body sick, sickness of the body makes the mind sick."

The invisible line between the mind and body in traditional medicine has always amazed me. As a Navy Hospital Corpsman I had my first look at neurology and psychiatry and how the mental "system" can and does affect both the mind and body in their health and functionality. The attitude of the patient often influences all other treatment efforts.

Throughout my journey in dealing with COPD, little, if anything was discussed with me regarding the "mind" part of the mind-body medical treatment. The mind-body connection was just left out of treatment discussions. Not one of the physicians I was treated by, including my pulmonologist, discussed the changes resulting from the effects of drugs and dealing with a chronic disability. I never made this important Mind-Body-Spirit connection in coping with COPD.

The mind, attitude, personality, and cognitive methods we use in coping were first introduced for my consideration in the support group session at pulmonary rehabilitation.

As indicated earlier, we spent one hour each week in this group discussing support issues. The remainder of the time, five hours, we worked on the physical aspects of COPD. Once again the priority in time allotment can be seen. After thousands of hours of consideration and practice, I think the treatment and healing necessary for the mind and spirit is equally important as the body. For wellness to occur the *whole* person affected by injury or illness must be treated

Katherine was an attractive woman, in her dress and manner. As a clinical social worker she had spent considerable time in the emergency room of a large metropolitan hospital where she became well experienced in COPD emergency treatment. She began to facilitate our support group by asking Fritz, Bob, Donna, Jean and I about how we felt in our dealings with disability and anxiety. She asked about depression and how it was manifested in our lives. We had not given these questions much thought.

Katherine invited our spouses and caregivers to join our group, which many did. We viewed videotapes about the mind-body connection. The tapes showed monks covering themselves with freezing wet sheets after which they would control their body warmth by meditation. We could actually see steam rising from the sheets as the monks controlled their blood flow for body warmth. It was evidence of the mind-body connection.

## Stress

The five of us in this beginning class of pulmonary rehabilitation also began to learn about each other. We began to define stress and understand that stress is a part of all our lives. We cannot avoid it. Stress is the nonspecific response of the body to any demand on it. There are three basic sources of stress: our environment, our body, and our thoughts.

Hans Selye writes in *The Stress of Life:*

*"No one can live without experiencing some degree of stress all the time . . . Stress is not necessarily bad for you; it is also the spice of life. For any emotion, any activity causes stress . . . the same stress which makes one person sick can be an invigorating experience for another."*

Every thought or emotion causes a molecular change in our bodies. These changes always cause some physical reactions.

External events such as retirement, deaths, holidays, and moving residences as well as internal events like thoughts of fear, depression, and anxiety can cause stress. The presence of the stress we are dealing with can easily be seen in both body and behavior awareness.

## *Body Awareness:*

Blushing, eye squinting, teary eyes, dryness of mouth, grinding teeth, shakiness, heart pounding, locked knees, rapid and shallow breathing, cowering, stiffness, turning away, crossing arms, putting hands on hips, etc.

## *Behavior Awareness:*

Increased smoking, accident proneness, impulsive behavior, yelling, blaming, inability to concentrate, increased eating, alcohol or drug abuse, increased use of medicines, headaches, etc.

We cannot adequately control the outside stimulus we are exposed to, therefore we must learn to control the inside "reaction" to it.

For many years I thought that I had to react to everything around me. I never thought much about it, I just reacted. We do not have any line or wire attached to us that directly links us to a thing or an event. It took me many years and I still work on being able to observe a person, activity, event, or stressor to independently look, think, and decide *how* I want to react or *if* I want to react at all.

During my careers in law enforcement and navy hospitals, I became a "reactor" to events. In dealing with an injury one reacts with treatment. In dealing with a crime, one reacts by beginning an investigation to learn what has happened or to stop a crime. It seems that we are more reaction driven rather than pro-action driven. Actually, one can and should choose if they should react at all.

During the late 1980's the sheriff's office began to be more proactive in our fight against crime. We started with major efforts of prevention on crime, drugs and driving under the influence, with community education of our prevention efforts. Unfortunately prevention programs took a back seat to funding. It was largely because "one cannot measure crime that does not occur" so it is difficult to market the effectiveness of prevention. We began to plot on a map with pins where crime was occurring in an attempt to predict where the next crime would occur. This proactive effort was very effective.

Remembering the above, I began to apply these concepts to dealing with stress prevention. We were learning how to cope by preventing stressful situations that would compromise our breathing safety by controlling the situation and further by controlling how we react to the situation itself. Again, *we can decide how and if we need to react at all.* By becoming proactive, I could minimize unnecessary reactions to things around me that had the potential to be breathing stressors. I concluded one of the reasons the "mind" part of the class takes a back seat in rehabilitation is  because once again, progress and effectiveness cannot be seen or measured as easily as body rehabilitation.

As I watched my new friends, I noticed that Jean, Donna, Bob and Fritz were not accustomed to sharing their personal thoughts in "group" feeling discussions. I could see that we naturally would need to build trusting relationships first. I decided I must give to receive and started sharing the frustrations I had learned to deal with as my disability progressed.

I finally noticed some supportive "nods" from my new friends and knew they were relating to my experiences. It became apparent that we had all been out of breath at one time or another and would learn together how to better deal with the tremendous anxiety that comes with it. Learning to relax and control our anxiety was our lesson. Some suggestions were to avoid stress-producing situations, exercise regularly, set aside time to relax often, and develop outside interests. In other words, take control of the situation, talk about it to others, pace yourself, exercise and relax. "But how?" I kept thinking.

I had tried with my "type-A" personality to avoid stress-producing situations.

It meant for me to avoid stress-producing people and toxic relationships in my life.

In a list of daily affirmations given to me by a friend, I read: "Keep only cheerful friends. The grouches will pull you down. If you really need a grouch, there are probably family members that will fill that need." Well it seemed to me, that withdrawing from some of these toxic people actually was causing me more stress than dealing with toxic aspects of the person. Sometimes when I stopped spending time in toxic relationships in which I filled an established role with some people, the result of the change brought more criticism and negative stress. This is especially true of unhealthy relationships.

The more I relaxed and became involved in outside interests, the less time I found I had to manage my disability which became more important than ever. In our rural town, many of the retired men had developed coffee klatches at different coffee shops. They were small, friendly little cliques of four to six men. Every day at 3:00 P.M. all would show up at the pre-selected spot. It was very socially fulfilling. I found that by having to be somewhere every day, in the middle of the afternoon, could interfere with just about any project. Other equally important interests can and did become demanding on the time that I was using to get to coffee each day.

All of this was making it more difficult to pace myself and accomplish the activities of daily living that I was already taking more time to do. "So how do I fit all this in?"

Once again, we need to prioritize our energy each day to bring the best results to our lives. Decide what you will do and when. Decide what you won't do and dare to say no. Try to avoid anything and anyone who truly wastes your time. By "wasting" I mean none of the people in company are getting anything out of the conversations or activity. Helping someone else is never a waste of time. For example, I have learned that my best exercise time on my treadmill is in the morning from 9 A.M. until around noon. I have learned if I do not do this important daily exercise at this time I most likely will not do it. I now guard this time tenaciously against intrusions.

Katherine began to show us "how" to prepare for these stress-reduction techniques by first:

Developing our relaxation skills
Finding a quiet, calm environment
Finding a mental focal point
Developing passive attitude
Finding a comfortable position

Much has been written on stress warning signs. The physical, behavioral, emotional and cognitive, spiritual, and relational symptoms are many. Each person may experience different stress symptoms and their intensity in different ways.

I was once told many years ago that stress was "cumulative" and our body is like a vessel or bucket filling up. Once we had accumulated too much stress without dealing with it, our stress bucket would "fill up and run over" as seen by severe symptoms. Stress signals explain irreversible burnout, and many other physical and mental symptoms. Many years later I recognized this burnout in myself. Burnout was a threatening change to me especially losing all interest in things and events that once excited me. I was disconcerted when my reactions began to change when confronted with things I had seen before as commonplace. I developed intolerance for violence after a lifetime working, without much reaction at all, in the presence of death, blood and mutilation. My bucket finally got full and ran over.

One of the best definitions of "stress" that I have understood I heard from Dr. Stan. Actually this definition came from Dr. Herbert Benson, M.D. It is said by them, *"Stress is the perception of a threat and the perception that an individual is unable to cope with that threat."*

This threat "perception" part of this explanation puts the reality into living stress. That is, what we perceive as a threat may not be a threat at all. Dr. Stan further explained, "The body has a built-in mechanism, the hypothalamus gland that secretes hormones as an antidote to prepare us for 'Fight or Flight'. Confront the stressor or retreat from it; this natural 'reaction' is to the 'action' of stimulus that gets us ready to deal with a perceived threat."

One of the rehabilitation patients that I was working with gave me this acronym: *FEAR = False Emotions Altering Reality.* This new understanding helps us understand that it is our perception that creates fear. This same perceived threat tells us that we cannot deal with it. What we need to change is our cognitive perception of both the validity of the threat and our ability to deal with it.

Current research shows that depression may be an illness that serves an evolutionary purpose as a useful way of protecting people from harm or from perceived threats.

As Katherine and later Dr. Stan and others spoke to us of the "Fight or Flight," first by the hypothalamus gland response then in our human behavior, I began for the first time to see the reason for exacerbated anxiety and stress in the COPD patient. Both a physical and mental change occurs with anxiety. We need to understand the literal preparation of our body to "fight" off this threat by giving us increased adrenalin, breathing, pulse, and the strength to do it. The same reaction occurs for us to choose the other option of "flight," to run fast and far to avoid the perceived threat.

Only with understanding can we then comprehend the often unrecognized and terrifying dilemma COPD and other disabled patients may face. *They cannot do either; fight or flight!* COPD patients, people with severe emphysema, not capable of breathing, and other physically disabled and compromised humans cannot fight or flight physically! *They get the anxiety but not the normal coping options.* Therefore, we must learn to "flight or escape mentally" instead of physically, on the "inside" by relying on relaxation and imagery to escape from the outside physical threat or stress.

I realized as Katherine was explaining this to us that we needed to learn how to short-circuit this fight or flight stress reaction. I could see that Jean and Donna were interested, Fritz was coming around, and Bob would wait and see. We now knew the most severe physical damage of lung disease cannot be repaired, but the psychological damage it does can be repaired and treated.

What happens to all that stress and anxiety when we cannot "fight or flight," or take charge of our thoughts, or develop new cognitive coping skills is interesting. It can be simply seen as a circular motion leading to a downward spiral of despair, which further perpetuates anxiety.

By visualizing a clock with twelve at the top labeled "stress," three o'clock labeled "automatic thoughts," six o'clock labeled "maladaptive behavior," and nine o'clock labeled "negative physical symptoms" you see a Negative Stress Cycle Diagram. Draw in circular motion arrows to the right (clockwise) and around the clock. This will depict the progression of stress to Negative Physical Symptoms such as "shortness of breath."

To make an Anxiety Breathlessness Cycle simply change the twelve o'clock label to "shortness of breath," two o'clock to "anxiety," four o'clock to "shallow breathing" six o'clock to "muscle tension," eight o'clock to "tiredness," nine o'clock to "less energy", and ten o'clock to "increased anxiety." You now find yourself back at twelve o'clock, which is "shortness of breath." This diagram drawn on paper makes it easy to see how we self-perpetuate our stress and subsequently shortness of breath. This cycle explains the chain of events with all shortness of breath and how the thought process can exacerbate the condition if not checked.

The Fear Dyspnea Cycle (progressing shortness of breath) is actually self-feeding. If we could slow down and listen to our thoughts as this happens, as the progression of anxiety occurs we may hear during the activities of walking, exercise, grooming, bathing, anxiety, social stress, depression and anxiety attacks the following self-talk; "I am breathless, getting worse, better slow down, stop or sit down, who is watching, more severe, less activity, fear of anxiety, it's happening to me again, where can I sit down, where is my medicine inhaler and how far is my help etc."

Many years after I completed pulmonary rehabilitation, Sally, a very helpful clinical social worker, and I co-facilitated a COPD Support Group. We explained this stress cycle concept while discussing automatic negative thoughts (ANTS). Negative thoughts cause behaviors that fulfill thoughts (a "self-fulfilling prophecy"), which justify more negative thoughts causing more negative behaviors justifying more negative thoughts. More negative behaviors cause a downward spiral to anxiety, anger, depression and isolation. Anger is a symptom of fear, most often of rejection, disapproval, or control.

The self-talk might sound like this: "I am too tired to do anything, can't do it, too hard, can't breathe, too many steps to exercise, I tried losing weight it didn't work, no one understands me or my disease, it's not fair, it is no use. I am not attractive anymore, I have a fat face, bruised skin, can't do the things I enjoy, no one likes me, it is easier just to stay home and watch

T.V. especially when I need my oxygen, no one calls me anyway . . . etc." These negative thoughts continue to manifest anger then frustration, fear, withdrawal, which eventually lead to isolation and a deeper depression.

These specific thoughts cause specific behaviors that contribute to COPD illness. This is a cognitive (negative thought) disorder. "Stinking thinking causes stinking feelings causes stinking behavior" (A.A.). We had to learn that to stop anxiety attacks it would be necessary to stop the thinking (fear) that caused the anxiety. By recognizing the automatic negative thoughts as "ANTS", Sally and I would suggest to the group we were helping to "shake off" negative thoughts as if they were ants (insect type). Like, "ants in your pants." Shake them off; get rid of them before they have a chance to bite you (affect you). At the very first recognition of negative thinking, get rid of the thought by replacing it with a more productive and of course, positive one. This exercise will help improve your feelings that will ultimately improve your behavior.

Grounded, well thought-out and validated thinking supports the feelings and constructive behavior we need in dealing with COPD or other chronic illness. Remember fear is the false emotion altering the reality of the threat.

From a workshop for the aging and the elderly, author unknown:

## The Eight Fears of Chronic Illnesses

1. The fear of loss of control:
   Separate immediate problems from longer-term problems.
   Make personal decisions whenever possible.
   Evaluate and change what is changeable.
   Pinpoint areas of stress.
   Salvage what you can from old coping strategies.
   Find a true confidant.
2. The fear of loss of self-image (internal view of one's self):
   List and grieve losses.

Let go of "stuff" that is no longer important.
Forge a new identity.
Seek support for change.

3. The fear of dependency:
    Experience the grieving process.
    Learn to ask for and receive support.
    Set reasonable and reachable independence goals.
    Give to others.
    Become involved in medical decisions.

4. The fear of stigma (external view caused by outside influences):
    Look at the world realistically.
    Reveal secret feelings to a confidant.
    Ignore disparagements.
    Remember, you are not your illness.

5. The fear of abandonment:
    Be cautious in interpreting family communication.
    Confront your fear before trying to conquer it.
    Discuss your fears with loved ones.
    Be sensitive to your family's needs.
    Remain emotionally involved.

6. The fear of expressing anger:
    Evaluate yourself.
    Expect anger to surface.
    Note where your rage is focused.
    Use words to express your feelings.
    Find a healthy place and manner to vent your emotions.

7. The fear of isolation:
    Prepare yourself for others' ignorance and discomfort.
    Ready a statement when your feel rejected or ignored.
    Let people know how you would like to be included.
    Decide how much support you need and want.
    Be realistic about friends and family.

8. The fear of death:
    Desensitize yourself to the fear of death.

Take charge of your fear by taking control of your life.

We must find meaningful reasons to live, not so much for more money, fame, contributions or recognition, but learning how to love and bring peace and beauty to our surroundings. This lesson has proven to lengthen one's life by diverting and preventing sickness of the mind and body.

I know and remember that worse than death is living without air; dying can be easy, living can be difficult. It is not about death, it is about living.

So we need to learn how to live. It is not *how long* one lives that count very much to me; it is how well one lives. We need to learn how to live well. I relish a good day because the next one may be not so good; so I get ready for both kinds of days. I call it "realistic expectations."

If my expectations are too high, especially of others, I need to modify them and decrease the chances of my disappointment. Disabilities seem to happen to us before we know how to cope with them. So how does one get ready to deal with a chronic disability in a more productive way? Katherine said she would show us.

I certainly knew what fighting and flying was about, I had literally done both much of my life. This was different; it was symbolic of how we deal with stressors or threats. This was mental work not physical and would require changes in my thoughts and feelings.

It was now a few weeks into our pulmonary rehabilitation class, this very first class for our medical center and the five of us with staff were experimenting with the new curriculum. We met once per week for our one-hour support group. We were still not sure what we needed to do in this group session. We may not have realized what a great opportunity it was for us to access professional help in recognizing distorted thinking and a chance to form lasting relationships based on our disabilities.

As I got to know Jean, Dottie, Bob and Fritz, I realized they were all very different people with different levels of formal education and experiences. What impressed me most was that none of these people complained much about their breathing disability.

Jean seemed to have accepted her breathing problems. She enjoyed her daughter and granddaughter, still traveled to different parts of the world never complaining much about the struggle it can be to make connections, move luggage, breathe the airplane air, pressurized cabins, changing altitudes, and avoiding people with colds who are a part of the traveling experience.

Bob was a quiet, soft-spoken, large man in his early eighties who had loved his game of college baseball. He walked with a cane, carried a smile for anyone, and quietly performed his exercises as best he could.

One day I was standing next to him as he exercised on the upper body exerciser. He had grown weak from corticosteroids and his skin had turned thin like tissue paper, a very common side effect of this medication that most of us had experienced. As Bob turned his hands and arms in a circular motion, one arm then the other, up and down, over and over, his hand brushed the top of the rough handle, tearing the skin on the top of his right hand. It appeared to be at least a three-inch laceration that would definitely need suturing. I called Diane the director and as we talked to Bob, he just smiled and followed us to the emergency room where they repaired his hand.

What a gentle man I thought; how many times I wondered, had he hurt himself farming and never missed a day's work?

Dottie, a widow, was a small, frail, blond lady in her early seventies. She had smoked like I had and simply trashed her lungs. She told me she had worked for many years on a rural postal delivery route near a beautiful resort lake. She had lived the last few years alone after losing her husband. Life was a struggle for her; she did not enjoy living alone and coping with her disability. Living alone was especially difficult with her breathing disability. Dottie decided to move into a small condo west of town where she waited for the weekends when she could see her daughter and granddaughter. It surprised me to see her daughter still smoked as she watched her mother struggle to breathe.

Fritz was a tall, thin man, who carried his shoulders high to ease his breathing. He had thinning red hair combed straight back, clear rimmed glasses and a gentle friendly nature. His wife was Ruby, an attractive woman with red hair, who worked very hard all her life to raise their three children and now their grandchildren. She was definitely his caregiver, as Janet was mine.

We were easily bonding as a group, both the patients and the attending spouses. We seemed to care about each other and looked forward to our group class. When one of us was missing we all became concerned and wanted to know if they were all right. We were now comfortable with each other and ready to share some personal information of how we lived with our COPD.

It was now time for us to learn the techniques of relaxation.

# Chapter 6

## Relaxation Techniques

### *Eliciting the Relaxation Response*

*The relaxation response is an innate physiological response of the hypothalamus that directly counters the fight-or-flight response of our body. It is a state of profound rest that can have a lasting effect throughout the day if practiced on a regular basis.*

Relaxation would require letting go physically, releasing muscles from habitual unconscious tension, and inviting the breath to become slow and even, letting go of tension with each breath out. To relax mentally, we must practice letting go of troubling and worrisome thoughts. Emotionally, we need to cultivate an attitude of greater balance. All of us can experience an enhanced ability to relax as we practice learned approaches to "letting go."

Katherine helped our class become familiar with some commonly used relaxation techniques that included:

> Meditation
> Diaphragmatic breathing
> Imagery
> Yoga stretching
> Progressive muscle relaxation
> Mindfulness
> Autogenic training

For certain people and certain sets of symptoms, one technique can work better than another. For many, a combination seems to work best and then becomes a part of their personal health regimen. For others, one or two techniques work best. As a person with severe COPD dealing with immediate and emergency breathing situations, I find one specific technique works best.

The most helpful lesson that I learned from relaxation responses was the use of "positive imagery" to cope with severe shortness of breath. I have talked to hundreds of people with COPD, who, once they mastered this calming exercise, used it to cope with shortness of breath panic, avoiding a trip to a hospital emergency room. Positive imagery is what I use to manage my frequent shortness of breath episodes with severe emphysema. Progressive muscle relaxation can also be used to help relax tense muscles from a bad breathing experience.

Sometimes I am not sure if the positive imagery leads me to better control of my breathing or if focusing on controlling my breathing leads me to a better control of imagery. Perhaps the focus is simultaneous as my hypothalamus gland takes over and calms my physical responses. I suppose it does not matter, but both focuses are critical for positive imagery to work. What really matters the most is to use the relaxation response techniques properly. One needs to be capable of controlling one's breathing. Practice by taking deep and slow breaths, exhale with pursed lips, quietly, slowly over and over while thinking "smell the rose, blow out the candle." The National Jewish Medical and Research Center also teach this technique. Pursed lip breathing in a slow, deep, quiet, controlled manner is essential for breathing recovery and better health.

Because breath is one of the only physiological functions that are both voluntary and involuntary, we can learn how to control the breathing process for purposes of better health. I began to see the relaxation response both as part of my treatment and as a life style change. This change in relaxation is enjoyable and calming to my normal, intense, type-A responses.

"Our breath is the bridge from our body to our mind. Breath

is aligned to both body and mind, and it alone is the tool which can bring them both together, illuminating both and bringing both peace and calm."

Thich Nhat Hanh, *The Miracle of Mindfulness:*

"Life is in the breath. He who half breathes, half lives." Proverb Imagery is synonymous with visualization and involves any or all internal experiences of memories, dreams, fantasies, and visions. Dorsey describes imagery as a "complex phenomenon of mind modulation." (Dorsey, 1988. *Clinical Training Manual for the Mind/Body Medicine Symptom Reduction Program.*)

## Positive Imagery (Guided Imagery/ Visualization)

On that day in pulmonary rehabilitation class with Jean, Dottie, Bob and Fritz, when we were first introduced to positive imagery, I fell asleep. It was December, the heat was on in the room, lights turned down, soft music playing as Katherine began to talk us through the exercise. As I was nodding off, my breathing deep, I felt relaxed. I could see in the seating circle across the room that Bob and Dottie were also asleep. Fritz and Jean had their eyes closed. This obviously relaxed state of our class was good, but "how will this work when I am struggling for the next breath?" I thought to myself, "Does the relaxation come before the controlled breath or does the breath get controlled before I can relax?"

The ideal and recommended setting for eliciting the relaxation responses is a quiet environment, comfortable position, and repetition of a simple mental focus and a passive mental attitude. The only one of these I have been able to focus on when in crises is the "repetition of a simple mental focus" and it is pursed lip breathing; *"smell the rose, blow out the candle"* as I search for a serene and calming image in my mind's eye.

I have found that positive imagery is most suited for my shortness of breath crises, but it may be different for everyone. In selecting what is right for you, you must think and remember a time and a place that was especially peaceful and impressed you so much you have never forgotten it. If you can remember the smells, sounds, tastes, and how the air felt on your skin and that it was powerfully positive and good in every way that may be the best image for you.

As I later helped facilitate this exercise for other COPD patients, I asked them to describe their image to me. Some outdoor enthusiast prefer the forest imagery. The serene forest works best for me. I take myself there mentally as I have seen it many times; starting with the deep green colors of the trees, grass, moss, leaves and ferns. I can visualize the grays of stones and rocks, the yellows of wild flowers, browns of the earth, and the gentle white caps on the blue greens of the fresh bubbling creek water.

Often, when I visualize looking up through the tall forest trees, rays of light can be seen shining down through the treetops like radiance from heaven. In the early morning I remember seeing a light steam coming from the warm dew moisture on the forest floor. I recall watching the movement of birds and small wildlife. I then focus on sounds and by slowing my breathing I can hear my heart beat allowing many other sounds to be heard. I visualize and hear the huge trees creak and move with the soft sound of the breeze. Bushes and shrubs rustle as the breeze touches them and squirrels and birds scurry from hiding place to hiding place. Shifting to the sense of smell, I focus on the sweetness of the fresh forest air. A bubbling brook or the rushing of clean creek water has a cool distinct smell of freshness. The pinesap and juniper trees have a fresh natural smell. If a campfire is present it really dominates my senses. Those who have hunted large game have experienced smelling the game before they actually see it. Our sense of smell largely determines our taste, and as I see, hear, and smell I can begin to taste the forest in my mouth. As I continue to focus I can recall the feel of the experience on my face. I can feel the cool air on my skin and my hair moving from a breeze.

Once we use all of our senses to recall this very positive image it gives us a place of safety and beauty to "let go."

It can actually take us from that stressful place to a mentally peaceful place, and it does not matter where we are, we can begin to relax. As we *smell the rose and blow out the candle*, our mind becomes calm and more capable of dealing with the panic of breathlessness.

On one of the occasions when I was assisting another COPD patient, I was asked "Is the ocean beach a good image to use?" I responded "If you can describe it for me using all your senses, it is probably good for you." She said she could remember seeing the ocean with its vastness of size and movement. The tides rolling in and out, white foam, greens, blues, and the browns of seaweed. She noticed the light-colored sand with ripples in its mounds from the sea breeze blowing on the beach. Occasionally she would notice a seagull first flying effortlessly into the wind then flapping downwind to build up speed. The birds would flock together and land on the beach near food or other objects, feet down, wings high, gracefully settling on the soft sand. She noticed the blue sky with a few wisps of white clouds floating or motionlessly hanging in a white puff. The horizon far away seemed flat and colorful at different times of the day. She remembered how bright red and orange the sky often was at sunset. She shifted her focus and could smell the salt in the air and the scent of the ocean foam and sea life.

She could smell a beach campfire and could hear the ocean tide roar. The seagulls could be heard screaming and the ocean air breeze could now be felt on her face and in her hair. She smelled her hand and could taste the salt from the surf air. She was serene as she visualized herself sitting watching what she had described. She had found a beautiful visual memory for her positive imagery.

I would later learn that the goal of Katherine's teaching was to affirm and develop a latent ability for natural and spontaneous relaxation response. Historical uses of imagery for healing, I would learn, have been to create relaxation to a state of sleepiness for treating illness. Simpler cultures have continued to use imagery for healing. It is currently returning as an alternative adjunctive practice to support and enhance medical treatment in our Western culture.

It is also important to use as many of the senses as possible, though everyone has a dominant order. Some are visual, others just "sense" images, and still others are very abstract. I included the senses of sound, taste, smell and touch of my experiences above. There may not be a "wrong" way; you will find your own image of relief from stress and shortness of breath. Mine works for me.

Here is another guided imagery for you that may help you find that visual "place." It is from the *Harvard Training Manual for MSR*. Katherine read it to our class. I have read it to many COPD patients. It goes like this:

Do a short body scan to relax all muscles in your feet, legs, body, arms, hands, and face. Focus on your diaphragmatic breathing. Sit or lie comfortably; let your mind focus.

Imagine that you are standing at the edge of a beautiful meadow. Let all of your senses become aware of your surroundings. What time of the year it is? What time of day? As you walk through the meadow, what do you see, flowers, birds, insects, and colors? What do your hear? Birds, the wind? What do you smell? The earth, flowers? What do you feel? The temperature? The wind? You notice that in the middle of the meadow is a beautiful hot air balloon. Look at the beautiful pattern of colors. As you walk up to it you realize that it is available for you to ride on. As you step into the basket you notice that on the floor are sandbags. Each sandbag has a writing on it. As you look closer, you realize that each sandbag represents some burden, stress or concern in your life; could be finances, health, relationship, job, or whatever.

Choose a burden bag you want to let go of, get the basket, pick up the appropriate sandbag and let go of it over the side. As you do so, the balloon gets lighter and lifts off the ground. If you want, pick up another sandbag representing something else you want to let go of and let it go over the side. The balloon rises more as it gets lighter and you notice that with each burden you let go of, you also start to feel lighter. Let go of as many sandbags as you wish. As the balloon gets lighter, so do you. You now begin to feel more relaxed and your mind becomes quiet. You float quietly among the clouds, drifting along, feeling content, peaceful and free of concern, enjoy this time of being quiet with yourself. Enjoy this quiet time for a while.

It is time to begin your journey back but remember, this is a special balloon and you don't have to pick up your burdens to return to the ground. The balloon slowly and gently returns to the meadow on its own.

As you return, remember how it felt to let go of certain burdens and concerns so you can repeat the experience when you feel burdened by these stressors in your every day life; gently step out of the balloon and begin to walk back through the meadow, again paying attention to the scene around you, focusing on the experience of the moment. As you reach the edge of the meadow, transition back into the room, opening your awareness to this environment. Open your eyes slowly stretch and begin to move, take a deep breath and connect with the energy around you.

## A Three-Legged Stool

By the time I was exposed to most of the physical and mind aspects of COPD and other chronic disabilities, I realized the interrelationships of the body more appropriately can be seen as truly a Mind-Body-Spirit connection. Before I finished my first year post-rehab, I began to understand that I needed a broader perspective of who and where I was compared to others. I began to see that a truly balanced, strong, supported foundation on which to build good health included the Mind-Body-Spirit.

I liken this balance to a three-legged stool. The flat round top on which we sit is supported equally by three legs, each one strong on its own but dependant on the other two. If just one leg fails in its strength or support, the entire stool fails. If all three-support legs are not fully developed the stool is unbalanced, unstable, not capable of doing the necessary job for which it was built. So it is with our human Mind-Body-Spirit stability.

This balance is needed for our human health, especially for the chronically ill or disabled. The balance necessary for good health is a healthy mind, body and spirit. The Mind is the attitude, feelings, and behavior. The Body is the physical condition, health and/or chronic disease or organ pathology. The soul is the spiritual, the Spirit and the way we view ourselves in the universe, which is a bigger and greater place than just our human individuality. Remember the word breath comes from Spirit.

## Spirit

I had been active in church worship many years ago and had "fallen away" from this weekly practice. I had married Janet who was a "cradle" Catholic and she gently and kindly urged me to attend mass with her. It was important to her, I thought, as I began to accompany her more often. I found myself looking forward to this hour of peace, sharing the experience with my wife and connecting to a "church community," both as an individual and as a married couple. This hour each week began to make a positive difference in my life.

I began attending some training classes on the doctrines of the Catholic church and ended up, somewhat to my surprise, making her Catholic church my own. This one-hour-a-week thinking of the world, the universe, rather than my isolated existence, has been useful to me. Putting myself and my disability in perspective as it relates to others with their own struggle has been very helpful in dealing with my problems. Focusing on helping others really opens your Spirit to healing. Connecting weekly with the "church community" helps me.

Whatever a person happens to believe or where they may find peace and an opportunity to reflect on who and how they are, it is necessary to develop the "Spirit" part of the Mind-Body-Spirit health and healing of the body.

For some it may be the mountain stream, the ocean beaches, a hilltop, or a place of worship. Wherever that spiritual place is, I urge you to spend one hour each week, without the interruptions of daily problems, reconnecting to that Spirit's purpose that is within each of us. It seems we are all really connected in some way. It is not as important "how" one maintains a weekly spiritual relationship, as it is to "do" it weekly to nurture your Spirit.

Knowing this is a personal issue with most people, I have carefully asked COPD patients who seem to be doing well, better than most, in maintaining a healthy attitude about life, if they spend at least an hour a week in this spiritual space. I was not surprised to learn that they did. Most, but not all, said they were connected to a "church community" and felt the support that it brought to them.

I frequently find new explanations from research that help me understand why we are all different in how we are affected by chronic disease. This article was recently available on the Internet and offers an explanation for the varying degrees of cognitive changes in COPD patients. In January 1998 I read from an Internet article: *Cognitive Decline in COPD Linked to Verbal Deficits* by Unmesh Kher. In *Medical Tribune*: Internist & Cardiologist Edition 39 (2) 1998 Jobson Healthcare Group "The decline in cognitive function observed in patients with chronic obstructive pulmonary disease (COPD) largely is due to the impairment of verbal memory, a new study suggests. Italian researchers report that both active recall and the passive recognition of learned material are compromised in stabilized hypoxic COPD patients. Only 20 percent of the COPD patients studied displayed normal verbal memory." Also, "while 38.1 percent of the patients displayed a group-specific profile, the patients of verbal-memory decline in the remaining patients displayed a high degree of individual variation," reported a team headed by Raffaele Incalzi, M.D. of Catholic University of the Sacred Heart in Rome. Published in *Chest* (1997; 112:1506-1513), "The study compared the overall cognitive function and verbal memory of 42 COPD patients between the ages of 70 and 80 years, with two groups of healthy people—one older, a second of the same average age—with a group of patients suffering from Alzheimer's disease."

This periodic Internet information regarding COPD is useful knowledge. I try not to over-react to what might develop with my COPD, instead I store it for future reference: Here is another article of interest: *Depression in People with Chronic Illness,* Duke University Feb. 2000.

*"Today we know that the link between depression and chronic illness is a two-way street. Chronic illnesses are depressing and the depression they cause often exacerbates the illness."* According to depression specialist, Arthur Rifkin, M.D., a psychiatrist at Albert Einstein Medical Center in New York, "The most common misconception about depression and chronic illness is that it's understandable to become depressed when faced with a chronic illness. It is understandable—but only during the initial adjustment period that should not last for more than a few months. Beyond that, persistent depression should be treated as a separate illness."

This is more good information to have stored in your mind, if needed for future reference. To manage our own disease, we must become as knowledgeable as possible about it.

In January 1997, we were completing the last few weeks in pulmonary rehabilitation. It had been a good holiday, one filled with renewed hope that I would learn new coping skills to live with my emphysema. Christmas was good for us in 1996 and we were ready to bring in the New Year, 1997. I was starting to lose the 55 pounds I had gained from taking prednisone. I had begun to wean off from prednisone and had discontinued my Theodur and Voltex without any effect on my breathing. I was getting stronger by the week. Now that we all were doing better on the exercise machines, we were increasing our exercise time to just less than one hour. None of us could believe the progress we were making and we all were doing better with the support of each other.

Jean, Dottie, Bob, Fritz and I were learning from each other in Katherine's support group as well. Diane and Wanda were supporting us through the physical conditioning, teaching us the aspects of lung disease, checking our oxygen levels as we exercised, timing us on each machine, taking blood pressures, pulses, and respirations as well as checking our perceived breathlessness after each exercise period.

Diane had arranged medical specialists to come each session as speakers. Some of these speakers were from the physical therapy department, the pharmacy who emphasized a pharmacist being a part of our treatment team, a dietician who taught us the correct foods to eat to minimize breathing problems and maximize the efficiency of our metabolism. Obesity is a real enemy to those of us with lung disease. Our compromised breathing system will not support extra weight.

We were even given helpful information on how to travel more easily with our disease. Dr. Ted, our program director, was also supporting this first program with interest. We were all seeing the results of our work.

In one of our support groups, Katherine brought to our attention.

## Cognitive Thought Distortions by Dr. D. Burns

Because it is so easy to begin to distort the way we think and once we adapt to it, it will feed itself into more self-defeating thought patterns. I include some of these below for your recognition and consideration:

### Some Cognitive Thought Distortions:

*All or Nothing:* (self-evaluation) Things are black or white, no in-between.

*Over-Generalization:* (An isolated experience generalized.)
  You see a negative event as a never-ending pattern of defeat.

*Mental Filter:* (Inability to see anything positive because you are too busy dwelling on the negative.) You pick out a single negative detail and dwell on it exclusively so that your vision of all reality becomes darkened, just like a drop of ink in a glass of water.

*Disqualifying the Positive:* (There is always a reason to devalue a compliment.) You reject positive experiences by insisting they don't count.

*Jumping to Conclusions:* (You predict what others are thinking and/or the future.) You automatically draw a negative conclusion even though there are no facts to support it. A friend may not say "hello", you decide they do not like you.

*Fortune Teller:* (You predict negative outcomes as a fait accompli, an accomplished, presumably irreversible deed or fact.) You decide not to ask a friend because they will say "No" anyway.

*Magnification:* (Catastrophizing or belittling) You exaggerate the importance of a negative event or mistake.

*Emotional Reasoning:* (You take your own words as gospel.) You assume your negative emotions affect the way things really are without facts.

*Should Statements:* (Unproductive self-statements) Accepting statements in your thinking like should, ought, must, etc., that result in feeling pressured, inadequate, and/or resentful.

*Labeling and Mislabeling:* (I'm a, She's a, He's a.) Over simplistic as in "If I eat a dish of ice cream I am a fat slob."

*Personalization:* (The Mother of Guilt) Even if something really isn't your fault or doing, you own it. Example: If your child fails, then it is your fault.

*Perfectionism:* You and others must be perfect all the time, and if you aren't or they are not, it is unacceptable.

*Approval Seeking:* All the significant people in your life must love and approve of you all the time; and if they don't, something is wrong with you.

*Self-Righteous:* People should always do what you think is right and if they don't, they are wrong and should be punished.

The above was adapted from Burns, D. *Feeling Good, The New Mood Therapy.* New York: New American Library, 1990. and Ellis, A. and Grieger, R. *Handbook of Rational-Emotive Therapy.* Volume 2. New York: Springer Publishing Co., 1996.

It seems at one time or another I have caught myself using

one of these "distorted thinking" examples to justify my thoughts. Have you? It is not important that we all have used these "rationalizations," it is only important that we recognize them and avoid letting them become a permanent part of the way we think and deal with our relationships.

Thinking in a distorted way can seriously impair the way we process new information. New information is needed to grow and develop especially to learn new and different ways of thinking in a disabled body and life style.

On January 21, 1997, I was presented, along with Jean, Dottie, Bob and Fritz, a Certificate of Completion of the Pulmonary Health and Rehabilitation from the Center for Mind-Body Medicine at our local medical center. On the certificate it is written: *"In recognition of your hard work, persistence, and willingness to make life style changes for a healthier and more fulfilling life."* I truly recognized this as the beginning, not the end of learning a new life style and how I viewed living life. I was a grateful patient and felt as if I owed our medical center a debt of thanks.

# Chapter 7

## Facing Mortality

Mortality: the condition of being mortal; death

*Learn that our time is limited; use it wisely.*

**Jean** was pleased and took her new strength and began to enjoy life in a new way. She traveled more and took her grandson with her to enjoy new places. We continued meeting monthly at our Better Breathers meetings and Jean was always a pleasure to see and visit about her travels. During the last five years, she progressively become more absent at our pulmonary activity gatherings.

Jean, her friend Sandy, Diane, her husband Paul, my Janet and I attended a theater play and dinner together. This had been Jean's idea as a group event. Jean enjoys the theater. She told me she stays home most of the time lately.

She is occasionally using her treadmill for exercise. We do not see her very often. Jean cancelled the last and only other time we planned to attend the theater.

**Bob** and his supportive wife Elaine appeared without fail to our Better Breathers meetings. Bob would occasionally exercise at the rehab center when he felt the urge. It was approximately a year later that Bob got very sick. I believe it was pneumonia that dragged him down to a frail state that he never again regained his strength enough to recover. I got to know Bob's son, John. John is a Franciscan Monk . . . he was there at my confirmation when I joined the Catholic Church. I felt close to him as a brother. Bob was admitted to a local care facility where I visited him the day before his death. We talked and I touched his hand to pray. He told me that he was "so tired."

In the next few years, I would hear this many times from failing COPD patients. I have learned that struggling for one's breath seems one of the most exhausting physical and mental demands on one's spirit. How true it is that "When you cannot breathe, nothing else matters." Bob told me that he was ready for eternal rest. In 1999 he got his rest. We sang "Take me out to the ballgame" at his funeral mass. We were friends. I miss him.

**Dottie** remained frail and kept trying to stay strong. She purchased a treadmill as I did. She told me she just did not use it and found it too difficult to exercise alone. Exercise seemed easier if she was with the rest of us or other people at rehab. Dottie gave her treadmill to her daughter, who told me she would plan to try it.

Diane had offered that once we paid the pulmonary rehabilitation program cost and completed the class we could return as many times as we wanted to attend classes. Dottie returned to the pulmonary rehabilitation program class three more times to use the program to get stronger. She was often irritable, confused, demanding, but we loved her and she cared very much for her first and only real support group.

Dottie enjoyed her new strength, took some trips with her daughter, bought a new bright purple Ford sedan and continued her struggle to stay in condition to breathe. Finally three years after rehab she needed full-time oxygen and began to avoid most exercise. That winter she got pneumonia and was admitted to the medical center. I spent some time visiting her and once took Fritz with me. Dottie fell, breaking her hip while at the medical center. She was using morphine the last time I visited her, talking about the past and how she loved to dance. She held my hand and told me how tired she was as she sighed in a low moan.

Dottie said in a moment of rational murmurs and babbles that she wanted to "just rest," and was tired of the struggle. The next day, we lost Dottie. She got her rest in 2000. Fritz and I never got to talk to her again; we lost her. She was my friend; I miss her, too.

**Fritz** and I were neighbors, we lived only two blocks from each other; I can see his house from mine. We became good friends; we visited each other with our wives every couple of weeks, played board games, and sipped some apricot brandy when we were not on antibiotics. We talked of old times and laughed at the way we remembered our town in the early 50's. My hometown was a boomtown during the construction of the dam. Like many small towns, ours exploded during the construction then declined after it was over. Fritz and I were here during that time. The 50's was a great time to be young.

It was post-World War II and after the Korean War. It was the beginning of rock and roll music. Fritz and I smoked Camel's and Lucky's to be cool.

After Fritz and I completed pulmonary rehab, he continued to exercise periodically. It seemed to me that he would never push himself very hard and would often have the wrong medication inhaler in his shirt pocket. I watched him use the inhaler wrong, sipping on it like hot tea, instead of as he was instructed. I never understood why. Fritz came back to retake the rehabilitation class three different times taking advantage of Diane's offer. Each time Fritz would get in a little better condition than he was, just enough to make his annual trip to Alaska to see his son.

For three years, Fritz made his annual summer trek to Alaska, completing rehab just in time to go, each time saying it was his last. The last time he went to Alaska was for his son's wedding. On one occasion Fritz exercised to prepare himself for Elk Camp. This annual event was to socialize one last time with his hunting buddies and grandson. It would later become a place for his memorial.

Fritz, Ruby, Janet, and I would sit at his kitchen table and play board games.

When playing board games that did not take much concentration, we could visit while playing. Fritz really enjoyed this company, mostly when he won. The last few times we played we began to notice that Fritz could no longer concentrate enough to complete his turn to play. We also noticed he stopped completing his daily and regularly played games of solitaire.

By this time Fritz was using supplemental oxygen, twenty-four hours daily. It had been a tough year for him. We met less and less; he just did not feel like doing much. His diabetes from corticosteroids was for some reason exacerbated. He had some trouble with his heart and had been rushed to a metropolitan hospital for emergency treatment. He was failing.

We joined Fritz with his family as they celebrated his 70th birthday party. It was fun. He attended the Better Breathers meetings less and less with me.

I would invite Fritz to ride with me to visit pulmonary patient friends but it got to be too much trouble for him, with his oxygen bottle or pack and he would decline. This final isolation of chronic pulmonary patients is common. I visited him weekly, would sometimes explain his medications to him and visited with his wife, Ruby. I would often relieve Ruby with respite care for Fritz so she could do her weekly shopping. Fritz started talking about dying and getting his affairs in order. He borrowed my tape recorder to record his family meeting, explaining how he wanted his remains disposed of and his business affairs handled.

One day, I felt like I could gently ask Fritz about our Catholic faith. He had been a Catholic all his life. The Catholic Church changed many practices during Vatican Council II in the mid-1960's, after which Fritz had chosen to stay away from the Church. I felt comfortable enough to give him my "three-legged stool" philosophy, especially the important leg of spirituality.

Fritz agreed it would be wise to get the "spiritual leg of his stool" stronger, and one day he asked me to call a priest. I did and he kept his word. He met my favorite priest, Father Jude. It was the beginning of the end.

Diane and I talked of Fritz's condition. We wondered why he had decided to give up; I think I know why. Fritz had talked to me many times about my cataract surgery. I had cataract surgery to implant a plastic replacement lens in my right eye and was waiting a few months to correct my left eye. One of the side effects from corticosteroids is the development of cataracts.

The word cataracts come from the word "waterfall," and with the development of cataracts, my vision actually was like looking at objects through a waterfall. It is indeed a blessing to have coped with the loss of vision through cataracts then to have them replaced with a plastic lens, take the bandage off and for the first time see magnificent colors. It is like going from black and white to technicolor when the sky, flowers, blues, greens, yellows, and whites become spectacular. After a while I got slowly accustomed to not seeing objects clearly and with much color. I did not realize what clarity I had gradually lost until I saw life with my new plastic lens. It is an experience to remember. Ophthalmologists must feel magic when they can see the difference they make in a person's life.

Fritz and I had this discussion and after continued reassurance he finally decided to get his first eye surgery and correct his vision loss from cataracts.

I stopped by his house the night before the surgery to share with him the magnificent surprise of color he would have the next day when the bandage came off. He never lived to experience this wonder of new vision. We lost Fritz early the next morning before his bandage was removed. He never got the surprise I promised.

Father Jude from our church and his wife Ruby asked me to participate in Fritz's Catholic funeral. I was honored and thankful that I had taken that opportunity a few months before to suggest to Fritz to strengthen the spiritual leg of his "three-legged stool." Fritz shared with me the last time I saw him that he, too, was tired of the fight to breathe. "I am really tired," he said.

Fritz and I spoke many times of losing our pulmonary classmates Bob and Dottie. It had been five years since that first day we all met in pulmonary rehabilitation; that time was gone; we had together felt the pain of losing them. Fritz was my friend, I was not ready to lose him, and I miss him.

During the last few years I have lost many of my pulmonary rehabilitation friends whom I often think about. I hope I made a positive difference in their lives, for they did in mine. The original five of us were special to each other.

*"A real connection with other people is rare and unusual, do not expect it with everyone you meet or know." Skip Fisher*

*"To the world, you may be one person; but to one person, you may be the world." Author unknown*

We do learn more from adversity than success. It seems through adversity we find and know ourselves. I learn through death as I learn from life. The death of my pulmonary rehab friends has taught me much about living life. Life really is about quality not quantity and not how "long", but how "well" we live it.

One piece of information that I always remember, perhaps because it is what I wanted to hear is; When we are without an adequate supply of oxygen, we become sleepy, relaxed and want to sleep.

I had heard this before as a commercial pilot; we were taught to use supplemental oxygen at an altitude over 10,000 feet. Those pilots who forgot this would hopefully notice a lack of oxygen before becoming sleepy and confused. It was further explained to me that it is not just the lack of oxygen, but also the accumulation of carbon dioxide that becomes lethal and fatal to us. It seems that it might be a peaceful death; one in which we might become sleepy, euphoric, and with the help of morphine, just go to sleep. I like this and remember it when I think of a suffocating death.

I also relearned that "tears happen." Endure, grieve, and move on. The only person who is with us our entire life is ourselves.

# Chapter 8

## Finding New Meaning in Life

*"I shall pass thru this world but once.*
*Any good that I can do, or any kindness that I can show,*
*let me do it now and not defer it.*
*For I shall not pass this way again."*

Stephen Grellet

I finished pulmonary rehabilitation with a sense of appreciation and new purpose. It was true that I was a few years younger than the others. My lung disease, the numbers indicating my normality, or lack thereof, was as bad or worse than the others in my class. My background was somewhat different in that it included some medical training and a life of serving others in one way or another. In both hospital and police work I saw people at their worst and somehow this has helped me through some tough times of my own. I had been volunteering at the hospital for a couple of years and knew of the rewards of feeling worthwhile and productive through volunteerism. So when Diane asked me if I would volunteer to help at the next few pulmonary rehabilitation classes, I was delighted. I was seeking activity to feel productive and regain and confirm my self-worth, a needed reform for the disabled.

For the next three years both Janet and I spent considerable volunteer hours at the medical center. I wanted to repay the medical center for what they had offered to me at rehabilitation when I needed it most. I spent two half days at rehab, took blood pressure and oxygen readings, helped with the exercise machines and eventually co-facilitated the medication management class. I was used as a frequent speaker at the pulmonary support group, orientation and graduation. I was also used as a visual aid as someone with damaged lungs at the smoking cessation classes.

Together, Janet and I volunteered over 1000 hours during these two years. I continued to volunteer in rehab and the transportation program while Janet helped maintain the medical center memorial garden. By 1999 Janet and I were recognized as "Volunteers of the Year" for the medical center.

In the spring of 1999 I was featured in the medical center quarterly publication, *Well Aware*. My success story of dealing with COPD was told. Diane and other staff at rehab and center for mind-body medicine called me the "Poster Boy of Pulmonary Rehab." By now I had painfully, and at the rate of one pound a week, lost fifty-five pounds. I was off prednisone, using a Flovent inhaler, exercising every day on my treadmill and had found a new quality of life.

This was now the way I wanted to live. I wanted to use my new strength. I would try to hide my disability. I seemed once again to be productive.

I continued to find medication improvements. New pulmonary medications are being developed each year and at this time Combivent inhalers, which combine Albuterol and Atrovent, came on the market. I got the first prescription written in our town and had it distributed to the pharmacy I was using. I was the first kid on the block to use it. Now I could carry one inhaler with me instead of two. When Flovent came on the market, I learned of it on the Internet and knew it would help me "get off" prednisone, and it did. Because of the three different dose strengths, Flovent could easily be tapered from 220 to 110 to 44 mcg. I had started using a nebulizer for my Albuterol and Atrovent four times daily. It works well for me and Medicare pays for the nebulizer medications.

I found a new meaning to life by helping others. I tried volunteering for our State Long-Term Care Ombudsman Program. After I completed the training and certification I began advocating for the elderly in nursing homes. I made two visits each week, saw every patient, wrote reports on neglect and abuse, and enjoyed advocating for the caring staff of caregivers as much as I did for the residents.

Each time I lost a resident through death I would learn more about living. Finally after being assigned to the Veterans Home with block-long corridors, I was no longer able to walk the distance and still have enough air capacity to talk. Rather than struggle with it, I left this rewarding volunteer work. In 1999 I received a Mid-Columbia Aging and Advocacy Award for the time and effort I had given to the elderly. It was another learning experience for me.

The Masonic order of Freemasonry is one of the oldest fraternities in our country. My great-grandfather, grandfather, and father had been Master Masons which qualify members to become Nobles of the Shrine. Although my father had talked about membership over the years, he really did not tell me much about Freemasonry. It was "secret," he would say. My mother had been involved in Eastern Star and Nile, which are also Masonic organizations. My dad died in 1993 and took all these secrets with him.

I realized in 1999 that if I wanted to know what my ancestors had experienced, I would need to experience it for myself. I wanted to accomplish this before the year 2000. In October of 1999 I applied to our local Masonic Lodge, completed the work necessary for the three Degrees; and completed the final work on December 13, 1999. I was a Master Mason before the clock struck midnight on our new millennium year 2000.

People really forget that COPD patients are sick even if they do not look sick. When they first see a person "completely out of air" they sometimes think this person is having a heart attack. I had secretly prayed that for God's sake if I was out of air that some old man would not grab me and start CPR, especially if he was a smoker.

I shifted my attention to Masonic Shrine membership. It seemed I could help support the Shrine Hospital for Children in Portland, Oregon. I learned more about this admirable philanthropy and how thousands of children each year are treated without charge for plastic and orthopedic corrective surgeries. It was here I learned a new lesson about disability. By watching the courage of crippled children and the strength it takes for corrective burn treatment I realized how insignificant my struggle had been.

I know a Masonic Brother who is a Shrine Clown and does professional hospital clowning. I was interested and wanted to experience the joy he seemed to be having. So I attended a clown training workshop and studied books on mime. I knew by choosing to do mime, that I could carry a stool as a prop with me and sit when I became breathless. Not having enough breathing air to do much activity, I thought it would work out well to do magic and mime acts. I bought and trained in applying makeup, bought an old black coat, top hat, and white gloves. I tagged along with my friend, "Friendly Freddie" the Clown, on his gigs to see what it was like and began to practice magic tricks.

## Unexpected Setbacks

*"One of the secrets of life is to make stepping-stones out of stumbling blocks." Jack Penn*

At one of the pulmonary rehabilitation graduation classes, I decided that I would try out my new mime skill and demonstrate how easily one could change from negative to positive. I carefully packed my disguise in a bag and went to the class as I had many times before with my famous graduation pep talk.

At exactly the right moment, I turned completely around in my chair, bent down to put on my disguise, white gloves and hat, and readied for my debut. When ready, I spun around to face the class and stood up.

What I forgot to do was breathe. My diaphragm had been compressed, seemed to cramp as it sometimes does, and when I was ready to perform, I had no air! I could not move, I knew I was in trouble. I quickly reverted to my rescue mode, as I once again started my well-known pursed lip breathing.

The "smell the rose, blow out the candle" act replaced my prepared mime act. It was frightening; I had to recover in front of all the people in the class. I had no choice; remember, when one cannot breath, nothing else matters. I did recover; Katherine thought it was great to demonstrate the recovery to the class. I think to this day she was just being kind, and my mime profession took a dive. Short-lived, but it was a new adventure I had tried. I did experience what my clown friend had and now know how hard clowns work to do the great job they do.

One other major "setback" to my progress surprised me because I was just not ready for it. I did not expect it; I was not listening to my mind-body-spirit. I was seemingly doing pretty well. As written before, I had completed pulmonary rehab, stabilized my weight, my medications, and was managing my disability. I had gotten involved in many activities that increased the level of my daily appointments and obligations. I was using the same two bronchodilators; same dose of inhaled corticosteroids and was not taking any new medications. I knew that my right eye had developed a cataract from steroids and would need eye surgery in approximately a year. I did notice the oncoming car lights in traffic at night "took on a star-bursting" glare, making it hard for me to see. Janet was a good nighttime driver and began driving for us after dark. It seemed I was once again in the mainstream of living a "normal" life, whatever that is with COPD. I was feeling a little pressured, but was enjoying the new pace.

I also noticed that occasionally while I was driving on the Interstate Highway near the Columbia River that I would "feel" nervous, and in curves near the water I felt as if I would "fall" which caused me to tense up. I put it out of my mind by ignoring these problem indicators from my mind-body.

I also began to notice for some reason when driving across bridges, being high over the water would make me nervous. One day, while I was driving a van over a high bridge spanning the

Columbia River, where the wind blows very hard, I noticed that I felt as if I would drive right off the bridge into the water. My hands tensed up, but I was somehow able to quickly recover and get across the bridge. I remained worried about this incident.

It was in late 1998; Janet and I had been to an event eighty miles away in Portland, a very major metropolitan area with numerous bridges and clover leaves on and off different freeways. The traffic is most often bumper-to-bumper and the exits on and off the freeways are critical to navigate and travel the area. It was just before dusk and on one of those evenings that the traffic was heavy. I was driving my Ford pickup, a Ranger 4x4, Janet was in the passenger's seat, the radio was playing some soft R&B, and we were on our way home.

I had just made an exit off a high freeway four-lane interchange into a sweeping turn onto a bridge lane that was taking us back down to the four-lane Interstate east bound and home.

I felt the tension start in the pit of my stomach and quickly move to my shoulders and arms. I noticed in my peripheral field of vision that I was moving as if in a funnel from four to two traffic lanes and could feel the sides of the roadway closing in on me as if I did not have enough room to get through. As I moved further and further down and around the curve I felt as if I was going to plunge over the side of the bridge. Tension was moving from my shoulders to my arms and into my hands. Both hands were now frozen like ice, with a death grip on the steering wheel, my knuckles were white with the grip, my body consumed with fear. I knew I was not going to be able to move the steering wheel with my hands as traffic was merging on both sides of us now. I thought of pulling over to the side of the freeway onto the shoulder of the roadway to regain control of myself but there was no shoulder on my lane and it was simply too far across three lanes of traffic to reach a place to pull off the road.

I became sick with fear and anxiety. Quickly and loudly I began begging, shouting, pleading for Janet to help me. At first I was trying to explain to her what was happening but the words would not come fast enough, I had no air to talk during the few microseconds I had left before I knew we were going to crash. "Take the wheel, quick!" I shouted. Janet tried, but I could not release my fear-frozen hands from the steering wheel.

Finally, only with the help of Janet and my guardian angel, we somehow got down and across the lanes to a place to stop on the shoulder of the road. As I sat there, shaking, nauseated, pursed lip breathing, *smell the rose, blow out the candle,* I was eventually able to explain to Janet my very first panic attack. It had been coming; I did not know what to do now.

I had a flashback of memory and remembered back thirty years to my days as a flight instructor teaching a new pilot to fly. I recalled the student that one day, through fear, had locked his hands on the stick during a landing near Palo Alto and would not let go. I relived that situation remembering the exact moment that I had to strike the student in the chest, to get the "control stick" from him, enabling me at the last minute to add full power, clean up the control flaps and abort the landing. Somehow we successfully took off, and climbed to 5,000 feet altitude so we could recover. I was now, many years later, myself recovering from the same level of anxiety.

I had handled many emergencies in my life, now I had my own and did not have a clue what was happening to me, but I knew it was bad. I later learned it was not uncommon for some COPD patients to experience "acrophobia," an abnormal fear of high places or other types of panic driven phobias. I was trying to learn if it might be caused by a distorted visual depth perception, spatial disorientation, medication side effects or even depression.

I let Janet drive the rest of the way home that day. I started avoiding all bridges and all roadways near water. This avoidance caused me to be trapped in my hometown. It became impossible for me to travel away from my little five-mile area. It was devastating. Janet began to do all the freeway driving. I traded in my new Ford pickup and bought a little Jeep Wrangler just for around town. I wanted no memories or recurrences of that panic attack.

I told my doctor, Dr. Brad about it the very next week. He mumbled something about depression caused panic attacks and asked if I wanted to try an anti-depressant medication. He offered to refer me to a psychologist that was good in working with panic attacks. I took the medication offer. He gave me Zoloft, which I tried for nine months without any apparent improvement with my acrophobia. I did notice some "blunting," dulling of emotions. I missed getting excited about fun stuff. I also noticed a lack of libido, sex interest, definitely a "fun stuff." The medication instructions indicated it would take a few months to notice the benefits. After nine months I slowly discontinued the use of Zoloft. I knew then I could no longer avoid this fear. I had to deal with it.

I happened to watch a television program one night featuring a person with a phobia; in this illustrated case, it was a fear of driving on the freeways.

It seems a psychologist was treating his phobic patients by reintroducing them to their false fear and actually desensitizing them to the object of the fear. This treatment was being used for phobias involving elevators, heights, driving, water and many other paralyzing fears. It was the information I needed. Janet would become my therapist I would become the patient.

It took many trips and trials, but over time, we would try many bridges, and curves; little by little I began to get though it. Remember . . . *Fear = False Emotions Altering Reality*. The fear was real to me, the threat was not. I knew that my immediate thoughts would be distorted. This would be one of those times, like my smoking addiction, when I could not trust the altered reality that my brain was thinking. I did conquer this fear as I had only once before following a plane crash. I had to fly again then, now I would drive again.

One day, over a year later, I was driving; Janet and I approached the same overpass bridge in Portland. It was dusk, traffic was bumper to bumper, soft R&B music was playing on our Jeep stereo, I approached the same "funnel" where four lanes of traffic merged into two, the feeling came to my stomach. I was determined to pass this final test. I began to *smell the rose and blow out the candle* through my pursed lips. I knew it was a "false emotions altering reality." I drove right through it, put on my turn signal, moved to the slow lane, and thanked my Janet for helping me get well and over this "stepping stone." I was now liberated! I now know how people feel when they are experiencing "panic attacks"; I have been there and back. I now try to help others with this unexplained and disabling part of COPD that some patients experience.

My first daily responsibility is to manage my disability, maximizing my quality of life.

*"Life is always about progress not perfection."* Skip Fisher

## New Meaning:

There are many ways that each of us can find to give our lives meaning. Each of us has different talents and special "gifts" to give to others. When I begin to feel isolated, limited and somehow deprived of a full life, I reach out with a focus on others and it is amazing medicine for my negative thoughts. Some of the ways that I reach out to others are by volunteering in meaningful activities and calling or visiting someone I have not seen or heard from for a while. The more meaning we can give to our lives the more reason there becomes to live. The more I have focused on others, the easier it has been for me to deal with my own disability. I want to have as many of these rewarding experiences as I can while I am still capable. I learned from watching death that I needed to live life to its fullest.

An example of focusing on others is when I finally got to participate in our local Shrine Screening Clinic. We screened and referred twenty-three children to the Shrine Hospital for Children in Portland for corrective surgery. I had seen this free medical service offered to children to repair burn scars and orthopedic deformities; now I could be part of it. This work taught me how others get through life with disabilities, many of them from birth. I have never seen such courage as these children have shown me in coping with their challenges. Many of them actually think it is normal for them to struggle with the activities of daily living.

It seemed I was looking for more and different ways I could give my life meaning, hopefully before I ran out of breath. In 2000 I was asked to chair our local Medical Center Health Foundation. Once again I was searching for meaningful work and learned this was a way to "make a difference" in community healthcare. By finding new ways to start and support numerous healthcare community programs we were actually making our part of the world a better place to live. There is no better medicine for us than to help others. It is returned to me ten times more than I can ever give. This Foundation has indeed been rewarding for me to be a part of.

Janet and I have become Eucharist Ministers in our Catholic church. We bring the Eucharist from our Catholic church to members living in the same nursing home that I had been an ombudsman in a few years before. This blessing does as much or more for "us" as it does for "others", probably more. This year I was elected to the parish council where I will get to serve with pride knowing that my church would trust me with this responsibility. This is yet another way to give my life meaning and purpose.

I am now afraid my time will end before I am finished with meaningful work that I can do. This is not for me to decide. In the meantime, I must monitor the level of my activity to avoid "over-committing" and "under performing", for I can no longer hide my limitations. I learned through some of these activities that it is necessary for us to see the thin line between being as knowledgeable as possible with our disease but at the same time not becoming consumed with it. Remember a balance is necessary among the three legs of the stool, the Mind-Body-Spirit.

I offer encouragement to those who seek new ways to give their lives meaning. As a "breathing-challenged" (politically correct) person, we can find ways to make a difference in our communities.

## Can or Can't?

Very sensitive questions that I have often considered are: *Do I want to be well? And what am I getting from others by being sick? What responsibilities am I able to avoid by being sick? Would I rather be well and take those responsibilities?*

I never expect anyone to answer these to me, but rather to themselves. The truth for some is they would rather be sick. It is sometimes a lot of work to function and deal with the responsibilities of an adult. Completing the demands of life such as working, preparing food for the family, cleaning a home, doing the laundry, shopping, mowing a lawn, washing a car, and all the other obligations can be exhausting for parents, spouses, employees or students that are not sick. I believe that before a person can get on a path of healing, they must consider these difficult questions. If the answer is you will get more out of life and from other people by being sick then you will remain sick, regardless of the treatment. The Mind and Spirit will keep the body sick.

One of the interesting paradoxes of lung disease is that we often do not look sick. When I first got my disabled parking permit and occasionally used it, I was either approached and/or scoffed at by some saying "You do not look disabled to me." I felt ashamed until I regained my composure and retorted, "Thank you, I try *not* to look disabled."

It was a long time before I realized the counter-paradox: If a person with lung disease does well one day, their friends and family may say "You are doing better" or "You are getting well" and expect you to do more. The more you try to do, the more trouble you may have trying to breathe. The more trouble you have, the less you will be able to do, the less you are able to do, the more they will accept you are sick. If they do not see you struggle it is hard for them to understand you are sick.

Shortly after joining the church, I thought I would attend a work party one weekend to install a lawn watering system in the cemetery adjoining the church property. All the men, women and children were helping with the project and I wanted to help.

I showed up that day at the cemetery to help and realized that I could not carry, dig, bend, inhale the pipe glue fumes, or do much of anything. I wondered, "Had my good intentions backfired on me?" "No." I went to the boss; he and I found something that I "could" do.

I used my car to get parts and supplies. One can see the dilemma and recognize that with a disability it must become what we "can" do, not what we "cannot" do.

I cannot wash my car or mow our lawn anymore. My Janet washes my car, and I help rinse with the hose. She mows the lawn and I service and clean the lawnmower. Neighbors of mine make remarks about me not doing our yard work. Those that have seen me crash know it is not a joke. It is about "failing" or "surviving." Are we a "victor" or a "victim"? Each of us can decide. Unless you try to do what you think you may not be able to do, you will not know what you can do! We must push until we can do no more to know what we are capable of doing. *Hence, the "paradox of lung disease."*

I write about this dilemma from my experience and hope it makes sense to you. It is true.

Here are more truisms sent to me by a very dear COPD friend on the Internet from Covina, California. She really struggles along each day helping others in a Better Breathers Program at Citrus Valley Medical Center. We do learn from each other and this gave me some food for thought:

> The most destructive habit is worry.
> The greatest joy is giving.
> The greatest loss is loss of self-respect.
> The most satisfying work is helping others.
> The ugliest personality trait is selfishness.
> The most endangered species is dedicated leaders.
> Our greatest natural resource is our youth.
> The greatest "shot in the arm" is encouragement.
> The greatest problem to overcome is fear.
> The most effective sleeping pill is peace of mind.

The most crippling failure disease is excuses.

The most powerful force in life is love.

The most dangerous pariah is a gossiper.

The world's most incredible computer is the brain.

The worst thing to be without is hope.

The deadliest weapon is the tongue.

The two most power-filled words are "I Can."

The greatest asset is faith.

The most worthless emotion is self-pity.

The most beautiful attire is a smile.

The most prized possession is integrity.

The most powerful channel of communication is prayer.

The most contagious spirit is enthusiasm.

# Chapter 9

## You and the Internet

*Tempora mutantur, et nos mutamur in illis.* 'Times are changing and we are changing with them.'

Static: having no motion, standing still

Dynamic: continuous change, progress

I have heard that all organisms in our system must "grow" and change or "die." Furthermore, this is the nature of most things. When we stop learning our information becomes obsolete. Computer Internet Web sites provide worldwide knowledge; knowledge is power, power that each of us need in dealing with COPD.

It appears that as technology moves us along in time that in some instances we must either "keep up" or get "left behind." Just because we are older is not a reason, limitation, or excuse for us not to become familiar with new available technology. This has been my observation with some of my COPD Colleagues regarding their willingness to learn about computers.

I reluctantly write this chapter because I am not a computer expert. Many computer users my age know more about them than I do. This chapter is written only in an attempt to introduce the computer, as an important resource that is available to COPD

131

patients to obtain badly needed knowledge. It is also a valuable resource to communicate with other lung patients of all ages and types. We are not alone and those that are "on-line" are never isolated; they literally have the world at their fingertips. If I've helped anyone discover this, then this chapter will have been well worth writing.

Because of my sixty-plus years of living, I have had the opportunity to see our world after a depression, and during World War II, Korea, Viet Nam and the Gulf Wars. I have seen the changes from industrialization to modernization and the communication information explosion of the 90's.

When I retired I had major computer programs and people who operated them. I did not know how. For communications, I used a pager, cell phone, mobile phone, two-way radios, three telephone answering machines for different locations and I still missed calls. I often said I was on an "electronic leash." It was a cultural shock to retire in the early 90's and relocate to a small rural town of 12,000. I quickly found that many of my new acquaintances in their sixties and older did not use a telephone answering device nor would they use mine. Much to my dismay, some would not leave a message on my phone service. If they were not home when I called, I would need to keep calling until I caught them home. I mention this, because as I became involved in committee work, it seemed impossible to do business.

When I decided in 1994 that the computer world was leaving me behind, it was because it seemed everywhere I did business a computer was involved. These observations included libraries, state employment offices, schools, colleges, banks, grocery stores, medical centers, hospitals and many utilities.

My granddaughter was learning and was very comfortable using computer games in kindergarten. I was intimidated. I was afraid I would *"break it"* when trying to use a computer. It seemed that when my wife and I took a few classes to help us get a start that we did not even understand the computer language. No one would take very much time to teach us . . . we would often hear "try it, you must use it to learn." I thought, no . . . I must learn, then use it . . . that was the way I was taught to learn how to use computers.

When I would talk about computers with people my age, they would most often reply, "Computers, no way, I haven't needed one before and I do not need one now!" or "It is a waste of money," or "I can not afford one," or "I do not need one," and other similar responses. I had said the same thing many times. One test I would use to strengthen my debate was:

"You say you use your computer to keep an appointment calendar and your checkbook. Pick a date next week and let's see who can check on it first." I would then flip open my "day-timer pocket calendar" and say, "See, I won, I don't need a computer." I would then flip open my checkbook and see the balance and say, "how fast can you check your balance? See, it is much faster for me not using a computer." Well, these are ridiculous examples and certainly an oversimplification of computer use.

It appeared simply from my observations that people from birth to age twenty were very computer literate; far too many ages sixty and older were computer illiterate. Why? I have wondered. I suspect that it is not the cost of a computer but maybe resistance to change, the fear of the unknown that causes this unfortunate rejection of technological advances.

Finally in 1994, my wife and I just bought a desk computer, put it in our little empty bedroom on a spare desk, and began to struggle along, learning from our mistakes. We experienced great anxiety when the screen went blank and eventually found a few computer people to help us. Some of these self-proclaimed experts are far too expensive; students in high school or college can be very helpful in teaching us about computers. We have learned to adapt and will forever leave the typewriter behind for this wonderful new word processing tool.

One of the most difficult parts of learning our computer was to become familiar with the "jargon" the nerds used. It was a strange new language.

Here are some words that help us "talk the talk" that I found in an *American Association of Retired Persons (AARP)* Bulletin.

**BBS:** A bulletin board system, which allows users to hold discussions and make announcements that others can read and respond to.

**Browser:** Software for bringing up and displaying Web pages. Two of the most commonly used browsers are Netscape Navigator and Microsoft Internet Explorer.

**E-Mail:** Electronic messages sent between or among computers that are stored until read or deleted.

**HTML:** Hyper Text Markup Language is the coding system for formatting Web pages.

**Home page:** The introductory page of a Web site.

**Hypertext:** Text that can be linked to other text by clicking with a mouse at designated points.

**Internet:** A collection of computer networks that are tied together into a massive worldwide electronic network.

**Modem:** A computer accessory that connects to a phone line and allows communication between computers.

**Password:** Letters or numerals adopted by an authorized user that allows access to locked systems.

**Search engine:** Programs that search any given set of documents for key words or phrases.

**SMTP:** Simple Mail Transfer Protocol governs the transmission of electronic mail through the Internet.

**URL:** Uniform Resource Locator is the Internet address of an Internet page. Each URL is unique, and there are millions of them.

**Usenet newsgroup:** Electronic discussion groups organized around topics of mutual interest to participants.

**Virus:** A destructive program that invades and infects other programs causing them to malfunction or self-destruct.

**WWW:** The World Wide Web is a network of electronic sites that are linked to form a global electronic network for transmitting information in text, graphics, audio or video formats.

**.com:** "dot-com," usually a commercial site identified by .com near the end of their web address. As in ABC.com.

**.org:** "dot-org" near the end of an address usually denotes a nonprofit group.

**.gov:** "dot-gov" near the end of an address denotes a government agency.

**.edu:** "dot-edu" near the end of an address denotes an educational entity.

**Case sensitive:** Some electronic addresses are "case sensitive" in that the use of upper case, capital letters or lower case, small letters, are specifically needed to make an address correct. Most addresses are not case sensitive and most often small letters; lower case is used.

**Important:** Every last letter, dot, space, slash, semicolon, and other characters in a web or e-mail address must be copied "exactly" correct or the communication cannot be delivered or found.

**Blue:** Letters that appear in the color blue indicate that by "double clicking" on the these letters it will take you to an address, Web site, or another article location.

**IMHO:** Used to abbreviate text: "In my humble opinion." There are many more abbreviations that each list uses to shorten the written text in e-mails.

Each year computer packages are offered at a better price. Computer technology improves so fast that most new computers are no longer new a few months after they are purchased. I foolishly waited to buy a computer for a year or two thinking I could get the "latest" model. All you can do as a consumer is buy as much as you can afford when you buy and know that you may want more in three to four years. Cost is based on size of capacity for data, random access memory (RAM), monitor screen size, speed as in Pentium 2, 3, & 4 and soon 5, compact disc (CD), sound, and many more features become available each year. You will eventually need a printer; someday most users get a scanner for photographs.

One can only choose what they like and buy what they can

afford. The decision between Macintosh and IBM is like the decision we once had to make between Beta and VHS . . . and someday the debate will end.

Most modern e-mail and word-processing program software now offer "Spell Check" and "Grammar Check" software programs. These helpful accessories will actually check your word spelling and use of grammar. If you happen to feel intimidated because of your writing skills, these program features help you write smarter. Some computer nerds write in all small letters and abbreviations that even make writing easier.

In the last five years so many "search engines" have been added that all one needs to do now is just type in a word and the engine will find a list of the requested subject or a list of Web sites.

A COPD patient today can sit in their home at their computer and just type the word COPD, emphysema, lung disease, or other similar subjects and access many available sites to learn about COPD and other lung diseases. I have literally visited hundreds of sites to learn about the anatomy, physiology, pathology, medications, treatments, and many other components of our disease. It is overwhelmingly easy. It is in fact much easier than using a library.

Electronic mail also opens an entire new world for people to communicate with others all over the world by "e-mail." This is especially useful learning from others how they cope with the disability of COPD. A "list" is a group of people who are "on-line" together. After joining a list, e-mails are then automatically sent to all the names on that list. A moderator manages the e-mails sent and enforces the necessary guidelines for the members of the group list. Some lists are over-managed and some are under-managed.

Early in 1994, there were only a few "COPD Lists" that we used to compare notes and learn from each other. I remember a few, such as Paul in San Francisco, Darcy in Virginia, and Peter in Seattle. Today there are many COPD "Lists" for lung patients to access. In addition to lung "lists," e-mail will enable one to keep in contact with their families, friends, and other loved ones regardless where they might be. Today many families create lists so each written communication is automatically sent to all members of the family on the list. It is a very efficient method to keep a group or family informed with valuable information.

Here is a list of Pulmonary Web Sites. There are many more, limited only by one's imagination:

Welcome to "cyberspace"; the super highway of information and communications.

http://pulmonarymedicine.medscape.com

http://gsk.ibreathe.com http://aarc.org (American Association for Respiratory Care)

American Association of Cardio & Pulmonary Rehabilitation

Daily Lung News site

The Pulmonary Paper

There are many available COPD lists and chat lines for written conversations.

"COPD," "EFFORTS," or "Emphysema" are other key words to search with.

# Chapter 10

## The Future Is Now

*"If you do not raise your eyes you will think that you are at the highest point."*

Antonio Porchia

My friend Skip who has spent considerable time volunteering to council people with disabilities while dealing with his own, once said: "If we live with one foot in the past and the other foot in the future we are then peeing on the present." I always had this visualization of a person standing on a gameboard with each foot in a well-marked spot named "past" and "future" while liquid dribble was splashing on a spot marked "present." This very visual image always kept me thinking about what I may be doing to my present.

I have been a worrier by nature. It seems I do far too much "what if," thinking for the good it may have served me in "being prepared" for whatever. By nature, and probably being raised by a perfectionist father, I was most often concentrating on the "destination" and "goal" rather than the meaningful "journey" or "experience" to get there. I am guilty of living too much of my life in the past and in the future instead of focusing on the present.

Since I have been forced to live with COPD and the severe emphysema that accompanies it, I needed to learn over and over that "when you cannot breathe, nothing else matters." When anyone cannot get enough air to breathe, everything else for those moments become secondary. Breath is number one! After a while, if you deal with shortness of breath long enough you will see. Just try to shower and get ready to go somewhere in a hurry and see if you can hurry. No Way! You can proceed only at the rate you can get air in your lungs. "The quality of your life depends on the quality of your next breath."

The reason this statement becomes so very important to us with COPD is that we really must live "in the moment." This moment of breathing, getting enough air to walk and talk is really all we can count on. Our present and future becomes *now while we have breath.*

I have always prided myself on being punctual and made everyone else miserable if they were not on time. Most of the time, within reason, I have learned it does not matter too much. Now being on time must be secondary and dependant on how well my breathing is. I always prided myself in a precise calendar of events, carefully writing each appointment on the appropriate day in the right space on my calendar. Since I have learned to deal with my COPD, I really never know for sure "what kind of breathing day" I may have when the appointment day arrives. Once again, my appointment becomes secondary and dependant on how my breathing is on the day of the appointment.

I spend the first and last hour of every day using my nebulizer. Early morning appointments keep me from my best time on the treadmill, and start my day off stressed and in a hurry. I try to avoid making early in the day appointments for this reason. During the winter months in the Northwest it can be very cold. I cannot breathe cold air so the daily temperatures become an important element in planning appointments. Because I never know when I plan to do an activity how I will be breathing on "that day," *my future becomes now.* One way that I deal with this breathing ambiguity is to respond to invitations or activity demands as . . . "I can probably make it," "I will try to be there," or "it depends on how I feel." I hate doing this; because of my obsessive personality I have always said "I will be there" and a person could always depend on seeing me. I have needed to change my attitude and remember to manage my chronic disability first then the other things in my life work better.

As I look to the future, I know that other "symptoms" may continue to require more coping adjustments and challenges for me. I recently read in *Breathe Well*, Autumn 2002, Vol. 6, No. 2, page 13 that:

"In addition to obvious concerns with breathing for people with COPD, the combination of too little oxygen and too much carbon dioxide in the blood stream may also have an impact on the brain, causing a variety of other health problems. These include *headache, sleeplessness, impaired mental ability, and irritability*." More than ever before, as I meet these coping challenges to maximize the quality in my life, I must remind myself that:

*My first daily responsibility is to manage my disability, maximizing my quality of life. Life is always about progress, not perfection.*

One other very favorite lesson my friend Skip passed on to me is:

*"What is, is and what isn't, isn't and that's it!"*
*Skip Fisher*

Once we can accept "what is" we can begin to accept "what isn't," and once we understand what works for us in our disabled physical state and what does not work for us, only then can we accept "that's it"!

It took me fifty years to learn that everyone may not connect with or like you. Heck, we start with a 50 percent chance of disagreement with anything we may say or do. It is "okay"! It is always about "who we are" and "what we do" that is important. It is a very interesting concept; if we do too well, some are jealous, envious and subversive toward us. If we do not do well enough for some, they are critical, condescending, and impatient with us. I always wonder how can one know how to please others when what you see is often not the "real" person?

There are some family relationships that are very toxic and stressful to live with. Some friends will never understand or even want to know about your disability. The dynamics of COPD are far too complicated for most to study or understand if they are not personally involved. As Skip said, "what is, is" and "that's it"!

It seems, for me, it is becoming less about the issue of COPD and more about how I think about it. In coping with a chronic disability we must realize and accept that we may not get much better physically, but we can get better psychologically at dealing with it.

One life style change that I must thoughtfully keep in balance is my vulnerability and frailty. During the winter months I must proactively avoid prolong exposure to cold air. A freeway flat tire on a winter night could turn a well-intended activity into a tragedy for me. Going down a long flight of stairs may create a bad situation when I cannot get up the same stairs to get to my car. Each step I take away from my safety and security means a step I must take to get back. I now must decide; is the activity worth the risk I am taking if I need to recover from an exacerbation of my breathing difficulty? I must try to stay positive, proactive and careful, but at the same time, "Do what I can and can what I try to do."

"Carpe Diem" means *come alive, on with the dance, eat, drink, and be merry as much as your breathing will allow you to.*

I have often mourned who I once was and the activities I could do physically. I know my beloved wife mourns some of the losses, too. We loved to dance, walk on the beach, and do projects together. We must never forget that our spouses suffer with us: we are one as an entity in marriage; what effects one in this partnership effects the other.

When I am down, Janet lives with me down and when I am excited, she must deal with that, too. It reminds me of Eric

Clapton's song, "Nobody Loves You When You're Down and Out."
Well, my Janet does!

The very first line of this book I wrote: "In mourning who we
were . . . we must realize who we have become . . . and accept
it"; this seems an appropriate line to conclude my thoughts. What
is, is, what isn't, isn't, and that's it!

# end

# Epilogue

*"What we have done for ourselves alone dies with us;
what we have done for others and the world remains
and is immortal."*
*Albert Pike*

I frequently ask myself, what can I do in the future to improve the quality of life for others who cope with COPD? While we wait for research and technology to find a cure or better treatment for COPD, and for those who feel like they cannot make a healthy difference, here is a way to affect our future:

It is indeed an appropriate epilogue:

## The Grateful Patient Program

While attending the Kaiser Institute Program on Philanthropy in Santa Fe, New Mexico, in June 2002, I gained a new appreciation for the development of futuristic thinking.

One of the programs that I became aware of at the Kaiser Institute, by Dr. Leland Kaiser was the *Grateful Patient Program*. My understanding of the program is that it is a very simple idea that can do much for our future COPD treatment.

The idea is to encourage *grateful patients* of treatment programs to perpetuate their gratefulness by bequeathing support to the future of the program for other patients. The insights, ideas, and inspirations we now have somehow need to be used to build our future.

Our healthcare needs are critical now, but will be even more so in the future. While volunteering in our Medical Center Health Foundation, I have had opportunities to see new healthcare programs, cutting edge medical technology, and specialized treatment programs offered locally to our small community by our medical center. I remember well that when I needed a pulmonary rehabilitation program I found it right here, five minutes away from my home. Also modern cardiac rehabilitation, diabetic centers, Plaintree hospital care and medical library resources are available. Most spectacular is our new Cancer Treatment Center, offering the most modern technology x-ray radiation cancer treatment.

We have and will continue to develop a more comprehensive Mind-Body-Medical Center offering even more advanced healthcare alternative options and opportunities in the next few years. So how did these programs get here? Who paid for them? And how was it possible? In most cases, medical centers, especially these days, do not have large capital budgets for such projects. The money usually comes from large endowment funds or estates that have gifted the medical foundation for specific causes. On occasions, of course, large loans are made. The philanthropy revelation to me was that it is not just about "contributing to," instead it is about "investing in" one's future community.

If someone had not provided pulmonary rehabilitation, mind-body programs here, then it would not have been here for me when I needed it. I live here; here is where I needed the help. I feel as if I have a debt and an obligation to assist in both keeping this program and other needed healthcare services for others. It seems to me that we have an obligation to develop and provide healthcare programs for our children and grandchildren, like our ancestors apparently have for us. It is the proper order of care and the nature of our progressive, healthy and civilized society. Each community has specific healthcare development responsibilities to their own communities. It will no longer just be the responsibility of the local hospital or medical center to provide every new healthcare program for the community. The residents of a community "get to" invest in this important healthcare function; they become partners and develop ownership in this important effort.

The first and last place each of us use in our lives is most likely our local hospital or medical center. This healthcare facility is the place to be born and to finally pass from this life. This is indeed true of you, your family, grandparents and grandchildren. Knowing this, in the future we will indeed want to invest in our life healthcare relationships. We will need to develop these lifelong relationships with our healthcare providers, as we have never done before.

This "healthcare relationship" will provide generation-to-generation healthcare starting at birth, inoculation, disease prevention, pediatric care, workers injury treatment, emergency care, community healthcare initiatives, school healthcare, pulmonary and cardiac rehabilitation, mind-body symptom reduction programs, as well as the final geriatric care needed in Assisted Living including nursing home facilities and finally, hospice, if needed. We need to develop a lifelong relationship with local healthcare facilities for our needed lifelong healthcare needs. This concept is grounded as it provides for our most basic needs. I have experienced this firsthand with my emphysema and the assistance I received in our local pulmonary rehabilitation program. I worry about how to keep the program available for others. This program changed the quality of my life locally, where I now enjoy better coping skills for my health.

One day, as I began to notice the obituaries in our daily local newspaper, I realized that many deceased patients that I had known and helped were treated in our local programs. Their families were requesting "donations be made on behalf of the deceased" to "The American Lung Association," "The American Heart Association," "The American Cancer Society" or other non-local medical healthcare organizations. The above organizations do great work for many people and there is of course a need to support them. *But* . . . I ask you to consider that if some resource funding is not kept locally then the needed healthcare will not be provided locally.

I admire the American Lung Association, but it was our local medical center pulmonary rehabilitation that helped many of us locally, including the people that have passed away.

Many of these *grateful patient's* families bequeathed badly needed money to national and state heart and lung associations forgetting to also support our local lung program that got them through their final lung disease treatment and many medically difficult years.

I advocate bequeathing some of the scarce contributed money to your local healthcare programs that also need the help to maintain and expand local treatment and rehabilitation programs.

These programs were there to help you, your family and friends when help was needed, and need to be there for others in your community in the future!

To implement such a program is almost effortless; just "ask." It is not at all inappropriate to mention this to patients in special treatment programs, especially to those patients who express "gratefulness" for the availability of such a program. A physician or other person who is suggesting the completion of a physician's directive can also mention it. I have seen a "light go on" in people's faces when I discuss this; they respond that, "it just never occurred to me." This is the exact response that I had when I first realized this natural opportunity to support a program that supported me.

It is easy to make this "giving opportunity" happen. Just plan to identify your favorite healthcare program and bequeath your available endowments and tax advantage property to your favorite healthcare program "through" your local health foundation. Consider it not giving "to" the foundation but "through" the foundation person or persons that you trust to manage your sacred investment for the purposes that you desire. Ask to see the foundation's receiving and giving policies.

Learn of specific ways that you can realize your passionate

dream programs now or after you have gone. Your favorite program may be pulmonary, cardiac, childbirth, geriatrics, disease prevention in the schools, or a number of other meaningful programs that will *help you help others*. Your investment in the community will live on to help others long after you are gone and will be "immortal." I have often wondered, "How can anything that improves my local hospital or medical center not be a medical resource improvement for me and my family?" Think about it.

> *"Never doubt that a small group of thoughtful committed people can change the world. Indeed, it is the only thing that ever has."*
>
> *Margaret Mead*